KU-533-303

LEEDS BECKETT UNIVERSITY
LIBRARY
DISCARDED

Leeds Metropolitan University

17 0125622 5

Principles and Practice Series

RESPIRATORY SUPPORT

Principles and Practice Series

RESPIRATORY SUPPORT

KEITH SYKES
Emeritus Professor,
Nuffield Department of Anaesthetics,
Supernumary Fellow, Pembroke College,
University of Oxford

Principles and Practice in Anaesthesia Series edited by

C E W HAHN
University Lecturer in Anaesthetics, University of Oxford, and Consultant
in Clinical Measurement, Oxford Radcliffe Hospital

and

A P ADAMS
Professor of Anaesthesia, Guy's Hospital, London

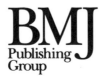
Publishing
Group

© BMJ Publishing Group 1995

All rights reserved. No part of this publication may be reproduced, stored in a retrieval
system, or transmitted, in any form or by any means, electronic, mechanical, photocopying,
recording and/or otherwise, without the prior written permission of the publishers.

First published in 1995
by the BMJ Publishing Group, BMA House, Tavistock Square,
London WC1H 9JR

British Library Cataloguing in Publication Data

A catalogue record for this book is available
from the British Library

ISBN 0-7279-0830-8 ✓

LEEDS BECKETT UNIVERSITY LIBRARY
DISCARDED

LEEDS METROPOLITAN
UNIVERSITY LIBRARY
1701256225
B41H
292525 29.995
112.95
616.2 SYK

DISCARDED
LEEDS ... UNIVERSITY

Typeset by Apek Typesetters Ltd., Nailsea, Bristol

Printed and bound in Great Britain by Latimer Trend, Plymouth

Contents

Preface

When I was asked to write this book I demurred on the grounds that I had recently retired from active clinical practice. In their response the editors pointed out, firstly, that my professional life had, almost exactly, encompassed the period of most active development of mechanical ventilation and, secondly, that I had been continuously involved with the design, testing, and use of ventilators throughout that time. When I realised that few had experienced the privilege of being so intimately associated with the development of this subject I relented, and this book is the result.

It is aimed at the trainee anaesthetist, intensivist, physician, or surgeon who has the responsibility for the care of patients who require some form of respiratory support. It is didactic and stresses the principles underlying the methods used to provide respiratory support, for it is upon these principles that future developments will be based. The subject continues to advance at a rapid rate, and details of techniques and apparatus would not only have obscured the fundamental principles but would have become rapidly out of date. Nevertheless, those who have read this book should have no difficulty in approaching any of the modern microprocessor controlled machines and understanding both the purpose of the controls and the logic behind the monitoring system.

Throughout this volume I have taken the liberty of adopting a historical approach. I have done so because I believe that this adds a perspective which is often helpful when considering the possible integration of new developments into clinical practice. In the historical sections I have picked out landmark references to illustrate how one person's idea became someone else's practice. However, in the rest of the text I have restricted references to reviews, or to those papers which provide further useful information on the topic.

It would be foolhardy for anyone no longer active in the field to provide didactic statements on clinical practice. I am fortunate in having two close colleagues who agreed to read the manuscript. One is Dr L Loh, who has had a lifelong experience in the field of neurological intensive care and non-invasive methods of respiratory support, and the other is Dr J D Young, who is actively involved in intensive care research and therapy. I have also been fortunate in having two sympathetic editors, who have not only made significant contributions to the development of this subject themselves but have also been close colleagues for many years. Their comments have proved invaluable and have been incorporated into the text. However, any residual errors are entirely of my own making.

Conversion factors, respiratory symbols, and abbreviations used in text

SI unit conversion factors

Pressure: 1 atmosphere = 101.325 kPa or 1013 mbar = 760 mmHg.
1 kPa = 7.5 mmHg ≏ 10 cm H_2O.

Respiratory symbols

V_T or V_E = tidal volume; $\dot{V}_E$ = minute volume; $\dot{V}_A$ = alveolar ventilation per minute

f = breathing frequency; bpm = breaths per minute

$\dot{V}_{CO_2}$ = carbon dioxide output per minute; $\dot{V}_{O_2}$ = oxygen consumption per minute

R = respiratory exchange ratio = $\dot{V}_{CO_2}/\dot{V}_{O_2}$ = 200/250 = 0.8 normally

BTPS = body temperature and ambient pressure, saturated with water vapour

STPD = standard temperature and pressure, dry (0°C, 101.325 kPa)

CaO_2, $Cc'O_2$, $C\bar{v}O_2$ = oxygen content of arterial, end pulmonary capillary, and mixed venous blood

F_IO_2 = fractional concentration of oxygen in inspired gas

P_IO_2 = partial pressure of oxygen in inspired gas (= F_IO_2 × barometric pressure − water vapour pressure = F_IO_2 × (101.33 − 6.26) = F_IO_2 × 95.07 at 37°C

P_AO_2 = partial pressure of oxygen in alveolar gas

P_ACO_2 = partial pressure of carbon dioxide in alveolar gas

PaO_2 = partial pressure of oxygen in arterial blood

$PaCO_2$ = partial pressure of carbon dioxide in arterial blood

$P\bar{v}O_2$ = partial pressure of oxygen in mixed venous blood

$A - aPO_2$ = alveolar to arterial oxygen tension difference

$\dot{Q}$ = blood flow per minute

$\dot{Q}_S$ = quantity of blood flowing through a shunt per minute

$\dot{Q}_T$ = cardiac output per minute

$\dot{Q}_S/\dot{Q}_T\%$ = percentage of cardiac output flowing through a shunt

V_D^{App}, V_D^{Anat}, V_D^{Alv} = apparatus, anatomical, and alveolar dead spaces
V_D^{Phys} or V_D^{P} = physiological dead space (anatomical + alveolar dead space)
V_D/V_T = (physiological) dead space/tidal volume ratio (normally < 0.3)
V/Q or $\dot{V}_A/\dot{Q}$ = ventilation/perfusion ratio

Other abbreviations

ARDS = adult respiratory distress syndrome
AMV = assisted mechanical ventilation
APRV = airway pressure release ventilation
BiPAP, BIPAP = biphasic positive airway pressure
CMV = controlled mechanical ventilation
CPAP = continuous positive airway pressure
CPPB = continuous positive pressure breathing
$ECCO_2R$ = extracorporeal CO_2 removal
ECMO = extracorporeal membrane oxygenation
EMMV = extended mandatory minute volume
FRC = functional residual capacity
HFCWO = high frequency chest wall oscillation
HFJV = high frequency jet ventilation
HFO = high frequency oscillation
HFPPV = high frequency positive pressure ventilation
HFV = high frequency ventilation
HME = heat and moisture exchanger
I : E = inspiration : expiration ratio
IMV = intermittent mandatory ventilation
INPV = intermittent "negative" pressure ventilation
IPPV = intermittent positive pressure ventilation
IPS = inspiratory pressure support
IRV = inverse ratio ventilation (inspiration longer than expiration)
MMV = mandatory minute volume
PEEP = positive end expiratory pressure
$PEEP_i$ = intrinsic, auto, or alveolar PEEP
SIMV = synchronised intermittent mandatory ventilation
SV = spontaneous ventilation

1 Development of techniques of respiratory support

Cyclical expansion of the lungs can be produced by generating an intermittent positive pressure in the trachea (intermittent positive pressure ventilation) or by applying an intermittent "negative" (subatmospheric) pressure around the chest wall (intermittent "negative" pressure ventilation). It was Vesalius who first showed that rhythmic inflation of the lungs could maintain life in open chest animals. In *De humani corporis fabrica* he wrote: "That life may in a manner of speaking be restored to the animal, an opening must be attempted in the trunk of the trachea, into which a tube of reed or cane should be put; you will then blow into this, so that the lung may rise again and the animal take in air. Indeed with a slight breath in the case of the living animal, the lung will swell to the full extent of the thoracic cavity, and the heart will become strong and exhibit a wondrous variety of motions."[1]

These experiments were repeated by Robert Hooke in London in 1664. At that time there was some doubt about the exact function of the lungs, some physicians believing that their main function was to remove body heat, while others contended that the motion of the lungs assisted the circulation of the blood. In 1667 Hooke disproved the latter hypothesis by making a large number of small holes in the surface of the lungs exposed at thoracotomy and then blowing a constant stream of air through the motionless lungs. The animal survived while the air flowed through the lungs, but it developed convulsions and died when the air flow was discontinued. Hooke also observed that the blood continued to flow through the lungs whether they were held inflated or allowed to collapse and concluded that the survival of the animal depended on the constant supply of fresh air and not the movement of the lungs.[2]

In 1776 John Hunter reported that in 1755 he had used a double bellows system to maintain life in an open chest animal.[3] These experiments led to the Royal Humane Society (founded in 1774) recommending the use of a bellows for the resuscitation of the apparently drowned. In 1827 the use of a bellows received a serious setback when Leroy reported a series of experiments showing that their use could result in severe barotrauma.[4] These criticisms, and the difficulties in achieving an airtight connection between the bellows and the trachea in the drowned victim, caused the method to fall into disuse.

1

The lungs can be inflated by:

Applying an intermittent positive pressure to the airway – IPPV

Applying an intermittent subatmospheric or "negative" pressure to the chest wall – INPV
- Tank ventilator: encloses the whole body with the exception of the head
- Cuirass ventilator: encloses the thorax and part of the abdomen
- Rocking bed: diaphragm moved by gravitational effects on abdominal contents
- Abdominal belt: compresses abdomen in expiration; inspiration due to passive recoil

---

Intermittent "negative" pressure ventilation

Interest then switched to ventilators that generated ventilation by producing an intermittent "negative" pressure around the chest (INPV).[5, 6] The body of the patient was placed in an airtight chamber with the head protruding through a neck seal and the pressure inside the chamber was intermittently reduced below atmospheric by the manual operation of a bellows or piston connected to the chamber. The earliest ventilator of this type, described by John Dalziel, a Scottish physician, in 1832, was used in attempts to resuscitate drowned or asphyxiated victims. A later American design by Alfred E Jones (1864) was used for the treatment of an extraordinary range of diseases which included "paralysis, neuralgia, seminal weakness and deafness." A number of similar machines were developed in other European countries but met with little success.

In 1924 Thunberg described the barospirator. This worked on an entirely different principle, for both the head and trunk of the subject were enclosed in a large metal chamber, gas exchange being achieved by the alternate compression and expansion of the air in the chamber and lungs. Although a number of cases of poisoning and poliomyelitis were treated in the machine in Scandinavia, the results did not encourage widespread use.[7]

The next major development occurred in 1929 when Philip Drinker of Boston described the "iron lung."[8] This was the first practical tank ventilator and variants of this machine were used to support ventilation in patients with neuromuscular paralysis due to poliomyelitis or the Guillain–Barré syndrome until the mid-1950s. The Drinker machines were very expensive and were not widely available outside the United States, but Drinker demonstrated his machine in England in 1931 and in 1934 Siebe, Gorman produced a similar machine for the British market.[6]

Several other devices were developed for the treatment of poliomyelitis at that time. One was the Bragg–Paul pulsator. This consisted of an inflatable band placed around the lower chest which compressed the chest when it was inflated during expiration, inspiration resulting from the elastic recoil of the chest wall.[9] Another was Eve's rocking bed, which utilised the movement of the abdominal contents resulting from the alternating head up and head down position to augment diaphragmatic activity.[10] There were also various types of cuirass ventilators. These consisted of a rigid shell which surrounded the anterior half of the chest, the edge of the shell being sealed to the chest wall. The interior of the shell was connected to a pump which generated an intermittent subatmospheric pressure to produce inflation.[6]

During the 1930s poliomyelitis epidemics were frequent, and in 1938 Lord Nuffield, realising that there was a great need for some form of ventilating device in the UK, turned to Robert Macintosh for advice. Macintosh, who had just been appointed to the first chair of anaesthetics at Oxford, made a film showing the various devices then available. After seeing this, Nuffield offered to present a tank ventilator to any hospital in the British Commonwealth that needed one. Fortunately, an Australian engineer called Both, who had developed a cheap tank ventilator which could be built from fibreboard, was visiting England at the time, and it was agreed that his machine should be built in Nuffield's Morris car factory in Oxford. By 1947 over 1700 machines had been built; 750 were donated to hospitals in Britain and the rest to hospitals in the Commonwealth.[11] They were used mainly for treating poliomyelitis, but in 1940 Macintosh also used this machine in an attempt to overcome the respiratory depression produced by opioid drugs during the first 24 hours after surgery.[12] As he later commented, neither patients nor surgeons took to the idea of waking up in a coffin!

By 1951 the existing Both ventilators were becoming unserviceable and a Ministry of Health working party was convened to consider the problem. A performance specification for a modified device was produced and the modifications were entrusted to Smith-Clarke, a retired motor engineer who at that time was advising the Birmingham Regional Hospital Board. He subsequently produced the Coventry series of tank ventilators.[13] These ventilators represented the peak of development of this type of machine, with tilt and rotation mechanisms, greatly improved access with "alligator" opening (a hinge at one end), and portholes and removable panels to permit physiotherapy and nursing care. Despite these advances the machines were bulky and expensive, and skilled nursing was required. The tank ventilator could be used very successfully to treat patients with poliomyelitis affecting only the spinal nerves, for such patients had normal laryngeal and pharyngeal reflexes and no artificial airway was required, the patient synchronising swallowing and phonation with the appropriate phase of respiration. However, when bulbar paralysis was present it was difficult to prevent aspiration of secretions because the neck seal made the use of a tracheostomy difficult. It was this problem which led to the switch to IPPV in 1952.

3

Intermittent positive pressure ventilation

The development of laryngoscopy and thoracic surgery at the turn of the century had reawakened interest in intermittent positive pressure ventilation (IPPV) but, although Green and Janeway had clearly shown the advantages of producing apnoea by hyperventilation[14] and a number of mechanical ventilators had been developed in Scandinavia and the United States,[15, 16] most thoracic surgery was performed by using insufflation or continuous positive pressure spontaneous breathing techniques.[17] In 1934 Frenckner in Sweden put forward strong arguments in favour of IPPV and described an automatic mechanical ventilator that was cycled by a device based on the flasher mechanism used in navigational buoys.[18] By 1940 Crafoord was able to report on the use of the commercial version of this machine (the Spiropulsator) for providing controlled ventilation during thoracic surgery,[19] but his demonstration of its use in the United States met with little enthusiasm.

Interest in the use of mechanical ventilation in Britain was aroused by Trier Moerch from Copenhagen, who reviewed the Scandinavian experience of controlled ventilation and described his own volume controlled ventilator at a meeting at the Royal Society of Medicine in 1947,[20] though Blease, an engineer in Liverpool, had developed and used his own ventilator in 1945.[21]

The 1952 Copenhagen poliomyelitis epidemic provided the major impetus to the widespread use of IPPV for long term ventilation. In that epidemic there was a high incidence of combined bulbar and spinal paralysis. Secretions accumulated in the pharynx and were aspirated into the lungs so that there was a high mortality due to pulmonary complications. A tracheostomy was required for aspiration of secretions but this was difficult to manage in the presence of the neck seal used on tank ventilators. Furthermore, there were not enough tank ventilators to treat all the patients. For these reasons Lassen, who ran the infectious diseases hospital, enlisted the help of Ibsen, an anaesthetist. Ibsen suggested that manual assisted ventilation should be provided with a Waters to-and-fro CO_2 absorber and a cuffed tracheostomy tube, the ventilation being maintained by relays of medical students. The results were dramatic, with a reduction in mortality in patients with severe bulbospinal paralysis from about 85% to less than 40%.[22]

Within a year, a number of new ventilators had been described and controlled mechanical ventilation (CMV) was being used not only to treat ventilatory failure in patients with paralytic diseases, but also to maintain adequate ventilation in patients undergoing anaesthesia with muscle relaxant drugs. By 1954 mechanical ventilation had been used in patients with severe tetanus treated by muscle relaxants,[23] and in 1955 Björk and Engström reported its use after thoracic surgery.[24] During the next decade CMV was used increasingly in treating patients with severe acute-on-chronic lung disease, asthma, aspiration and other forms of pneumonia, pulmonary

4

oedema, and the postoperative chest complications after cardiac surgery.[25] There was, however, one major difference between the technique used in the United States and the Scandinavian and British practice, and that was that American units tended to use ventilators such as the Bird and the Bennett, which delivered a breath when triggered by the patient (assisted mechanical ventilation; AMV), while the Europeans rarely used patient triggering and relied on hyperventilation and sedative or muscle relaxant drugs to maintain control of ventilation. Only in the past two decades have improvements in patient triggering devices resulted in their use throughout Europe.

The treatment of acute lung disease

The next major advance was the recognition that lung compliance (a measure of lung distensibility) was reduced in patients who had severe acute lung disease with consolidation, collapse, or pulmonary oedema. As a result, adequate alveolar ventilation could be maintained only by the use of high inflation pressures. Functional residual capacity (the volume of gas in the lungs at the end of a normal expiration) was also decreased, and this was associated with a decrease in arterial PO_2 due to the increased intrapulmonary shunt. In 1967 Ashbaugh and colleagues described the profound arterial hypoxaemia and pathological changes in the lung that characterised the adult respiratory distress syndrome (ARDS) and reported that arterial PO_2 could be increased by adding a positive end expiratory pressure (PEEP) to increase end expiratory lung volume during mechanical ventilation.[26]

By 1970 it had become clear that the addition of a positive end expiratory pressure resulted in a further increase in peak and mean airway pressures and an increased incidence of pulmonary barotrauma.[27] The increased pressures were also transmitted to the pulmonary circulation and pleural space and so decreased cardiac output. The reduction in output decreased the total quantity of oxygen delivered to the tissues per minute, thus tending to offset the beneficial effects resulting from the increase in arterial PO_2 produced by the PEEP. During the next 10 years several different strategies were evolved in an attempt to minimise these effects.

Minimising the reduction in cardiac output

It was soon recognised that the reduction in cardiac output produced by applying PEEP was due mainly to the decreased venous return resulting from the increase in mean intrathoracic pressure. Two approaches were used to overcome this problem. The first was to increase central venous pressure, and the second was to minimise the increase in mean intrathoracic pressure by allowing the patient to breathe spontaneously for part or all of the time, the spontaneous ventilation then being augmented by "mandatory" breaths from the ventilator at appropriate intervals.

5

Methods of reducing circulatory effects of positive end expiratory pressure

Increase central venous pressure:
  Raise the legs
  Apply an antigravity suit
  Increase blood volume
  Infuse venoconstrictor drugs

Reduce mean intrathoracic pressure by maximising spontaneous breathing component of support mode:
  Continuous positive pressure breathing – CPAP or CPPB
  Intermittent mandatory ventilation – IMV
  Synchronised intermittent mandatory ventilation – SIMV
  Mandatory minute volume – MMV
  Inspiratory pressure support – IPS
  Airway pressure release ventilation – APRV
  Biphasic positive pressure ventilation – BIPAP

Increasing venous return. Although attempts were made to increase central venous pressure by elevation of the legs or the application of an antigravity suit, most clinicians soon found that better control was obtained by increasing blood volume[28, 29] or by giving vasoconstrictor drugs.[30] Although an increase in venous pressure may decrease lymph drainage through the thoracic duct and may have other deleterious effects, it provides a useful method of minimising the decrease in cardiac output when high airway pressures are required. In patients with cardiac disease, however, right and left heart filling pressures may differ, so blood volume adjustments made on the basis of central venous pressure measurements may not result in optimal left ventricular filling pressures.

The introduction, in 1970, of balloon tipped pulmonary artery catheters[31] revolutionised patient care by enabling clinicians to determine the relation between cardiac output, measured by thermodilution techniques, and left heart filling pressures. Although it is now common practice to optimise cardiac output by manipulating blood volume, vasomotor tone, and inotropic support, there is unfortunately little evidence that the use of pulmonary artery catheters is associated with any decrease in mortality. Indeed, the converse may be true.[32]

Techniques that reduce mean intrathoracic pressure. The second approach to the circulatory problem was to utilise ventilatory techniques that minimised the increase in intrathoracic pressure by permitting spontaneous breathing between the controlled breaths. The lowest mean intrathoracic pressure for a given increase in end expiratory lung volume is achieved by using continuous

6

positive airway pressure breathing (CPAP or CPPB) without the addition of any mechanically assisted breaths. This technique originated from Barach's observation that, in patients with chronic obstructive airways disease, expiration was facilitated by breathing out through pursed lips. Barach initially used positive airway pressure breathing to improve gas exchange during the administration of helium-oxygen mixtures to patients with asthma, and later applied the technique to the treatment of pulmonary oedema and other lung conditions. The technique was further developed to enable airmen to fly at high altitude during the second world war, and after the war it was used sporadically in chest medicine.[33]

In 1970 Gregory advocated the use of continuous positive pressure breathing for the treatment of neonatal respiratory distress.[34] Its successful use in adults was reported two years later.[35]

Continuous positive pressure breathing improves oxygenation but does not assist CO_2 elimination and, in a number of patients, depression of the respiratory centre by sedative drugs or progression of the disease process results in an increased PCO_2 and the need for ventilatory assistance. Initially, this was provided by controlled mechanical ventilation; however, within a few years several techniques which combined spontaneous and controlled ventilation had been developed.

The first of these techniques was intermittent mandatory ventilation (IMV). This originated in paediatric practice, where it was difficult to achieve effective patient triggering of the ventilator because of the small spontaneous tidal volumes. The first IMV circuit was incorporated in the Baby Bird ventilator,[36] and in 1973 the method was recommended as a means of weaning adults from a ventilator.[37] During IMV the low frequency "mandatory" breaths delivered by the ventilator were superimposed on the patient's spontaneous breathing pattern, no attempt being made to synchronise the mandatory breath with a spontaneous breath. Initially, separate breathing systems were used to provide the respired gases for the mandatory and spontaneous breaths, but later ventilators incorporated IMV facilities within a common breathing system.

Manufacturers subsequently introduced ventilators that were capable of synchronising the mandatory breath with one of the patient's spontaneous breaths (synchronised intermittent mandatory ventilation; SIMV). To prevent the occurrence of a mandatory breath with every spontaneous breath (the pattern seen with patient triggered or assisted mechanical ventilation), the ventilator generated a timing window at preset intervals. The frequency and duration of this window could be adjusted by the operator, and the mechanism was arranged so that a mandatory breath could be triggered by a spontaneous breath only if it occurred during this period. Most ventilators had a backup mechanism that delivered a mandatory breath if the trigger had not been activated within a given time.

A further degree of sophistication was provided by the concept of

7

mandatory minute volume (MMV).[38] This enabled the operator to select a minute volume that was considered appropriate for the patient's needs: if the patient failed to achieve this volume when breathing spontaneously, the ventilator would provide the balance. In most ventilators the deficiency in minute volume is corrected by adding additional mandatory breaths at appropriate intervals. In one of the latest machines, however, the patient's ventilation is monitored continuously, and if the minute volume falls below an acceptable level, the ventilator delivers an appropriate pressure to the airway to augment each spontaneous breath so that the preset minute volume is achieved. This is really an automated form of inspiratory pressure support.

The technique of inspiratory pressure support (IPS) was introduced in the mid-1980s. The major difference between inspiratory pressure support and all the previously used patient triggered modalities is that the ventilator generates a preset pattern of pressure during inspiration rather than a preset pattern of flow. The inspiratory pressure augments the patient's spontaneous respiratory muscle activity so that the patient can largely determine the pattern of each breath, whereas with the other patient triggered modes the pattern of breath is determined mainly by the setting of the controls on the ventilator.[39] The level of pressure support may be low (just sufficient to overcome the resistance of the tubes and airways) or may be high enough to almost completely eliminate the work of breathing. In either event, it is the patient who controls the pattern of breathing, inspiration usually being terminated when inspiratory flow decreases to a preset level, such as 25% of the peak flow. To increase safety, inspiration may also be terminated after a preset time or if the airway pressure exceeds a preset limit.

Reducing peak airway pressure

The second area of concern resulting from the introduction of positive end expiratory pressure was that it resulted in a similar increase in peak inspiratory pressure, and so tended to increase the frequency of air leaks from the lung. Subsequently, it was recognised that the high airway pressures caused overdistension of ventilated areas of lung, which led to pulmonary capillary damage and pathological changes similar to those seen in the early stages of the adult respiratory distress syndrome. This led to attempts to reduce peak airway pressures. The most obvious way of achieving this is to increase the frequency of ventilation so that tidal volume can be reduced. A second way is to reduce alveolar dead space by prolonging inspiration; a third is to assist gas exchange with an artificial lung.

High frequency ventilation. High frequency ventilation (HFV), which is usually defined as ventilation at more than three times the natural breathing frequency, was introduced in the early 1970s.[40] There are basically three techniques. The first to be used was high frequency positive pressure

Methods of reducing peak airway pressure

- High frequency ventilation – HFV
    High frequency positive pressure ventilation – HFPPV
    High frequency jet ventilation – HFJV
    High frequency oscillation – HFO
- Inverse ratio ventilation – IRV
- Airway pressure release ventilation – APRV
- Biphasic positive pressure ventilation – BIPAP
- Extracorporeal gas exchange
    Extracorporeal membrane oxygenation – ECMO
    Extracorporeal CO_2 removal – $ECCO_2R$
- Intravascular gas exchange

ventilation (HFPPV), in which pulses of gas were delivered through a narrow, rigid tube directly into the trachea so that dead space and compressible volume were at a minimum. There was no entrainment of other gas, and expiration was passive. HFPPV could also be provided by directing a constant flow of gas into a T piece system, expiration being controlled with a mechanically operated expiratory valve.

The second technique, which has been widely used in clinical practice, is high frequency jet ventilation. A jet of gas is generated by a high pressure gas source and interrupted at frequencies of 1–5 Hz. The jet issues from a narrow tube (1–2 mm internal diameter) and then entrains a variable amount of ambient gas, the lungs being inflated by the pressure generated by the pulse of gas. Expiration is passive. The tip of the jet tube may be placed in the pharynx or inserted into the trachea through the larynx or cricothyroid membrane, but for long term use the jet tube is incorporated into the wall of a special cuffed endotracheal tube.

The increase in respiratory frequency allows tidal volume and peak inspiratory pressure to be decreased, but studies have shown that physiological dead space does not decrease in proportion to tidal volume, so that there is an approximately linear increase in minute volume with increase in frequency. Since the increase in frequency results in an increase in minute volume, and since the proportion of each minute devoted to inspiration does not change, there must be an increase in flow rate with frequency. At frequencies of 60–100 breaths/min, flow rates may be in the region of 20–100 per minute. It is extremely difficult to humidify the inspired gas at such high flow rates, and so rapid cooling of the patient may occur.

Two controlled trials of this technique in patients with ARDS failed to show any improvement in mortality,[41, 42] so the use of the technique is now generally restricted to specific situations where it is necessary to provide ventilation in the presence of an open airway. Examples are larygeal surgery, laser surgery of the trachea, and tracheal reconstruction. The transtracheal delivery of the jet through a 14 gauge cannula (2 mm internal diameter) may prove life saving when there are difficulties with tracheal intubation.

The third type of high frequency ventilation is high frequency oscillation (HFO). Because of the high power required this has been used mainly in neonates. A small piston pump oscillates gas between the alveoli and a bias flow of fresh gas, which crosses the outer end of the tracheal tube. It is claimed that at frequencies of 5–30 Hz adequate gas exchange can be achieved with tidal volumes less than the dead space, but measurements at high frequencies are subject to error, and there are grounds for believing that the volume of gas entering or leaving the alveoli may be smaller or greater than the stroke of the pump, depending on the local conditions. The success of the technique depends on the recruitment of collapsed areas of lung by a slow hyperinflation and the subsequent maintenance of the lung at the high volume by the increase in mean alveolar pressure generated by the oscillations. Although there have been some encouraging clinical reports, the only (poorly designed) controlled trial failed to show any advantages of the technique when compared with conventional methods of treatment.[43, 44]

It has recently been reported that the application of high frequency oscillations to the chest wall increases CO_2 elimination in spontaneously breathing patients. However, it is not yet clear whether this technique will prove useful in clinical practice.

Inverse ratio ventilation. The second method of reducing peak pressure, the use of an increased duration of inspiration (which has become known as inverse ratio ventilation; IRV), was introduced by paediatricians in an attempt to reduce lung damage and improve oxygenation in babies with the neonatal respiratory distress syndrome.[45] It was reasoned that the prolonged duration of inspiration would prolong the time during which the alveoli were held open and so would improve gas exchange. Subsequent studies in adults showed that the delayed emptying of the lung increased the efficiency of CO_2 elimination so that minute volume could be reduced by 10–15%, while the short expiratory period generated a positive pressure in the alveoli which decreased the intrapulmonary shunt.[46]

A similar airway pressure pattern to IRV is generated during airway pressure release ventilation (APRV) but the patient breathes spontaneously throughout the cycle.[47] The patient breathes through a continuous positive airway pressure breathing system, but the system is then opened to atmosphere for 1–2 seconds at regular intervals by opening a second valve. The lung deflates when exposed to atmospheric pressure and is then re-inflated when CPAP is re-established by closing the second valve. This technique minimises peak airway pressure but each deflation to atmospheric pressure augments CO_2 elimination. A recent modification of this technique is BIPAP (biphasic positive airway pressure), in which the patient breathes spontaneously at two different levels of CPAP, the levels being varied at slow respiratory frequencies.[48]

Artificial lungs. Finally, mention must be made of techniques of maintaining gas exchange by the use of an artificial lung. The earliest attempts at extracorporeal membrane oxygenation (ECMO) utilised a venoarterial extracorporeal circuit similar to that used in open heart surgery, so that all the cardiac output had to flow through the membrane lung. The need for heparinisation led to considerable blood loss from cannulation sites, and the high flows resulted in haemolysis, a reduction in platelet count, and the need for a high level of supervision. A controlled trial failed to show any reduction in mortality in comparison with conventional ventilator treatment.[49] However, this technique has subsequently proved of great value in some forms of neonatal respiratory distress,[50] though there is some concern with potential neurological damage from the cannulation of the carotid artery.

In 1978 Kolobow and others suggested that improved results could be obtained by separating the processes of oxygen uptake and carbon dioxide removal.[51] They showed experimentally that the total CO_2 production could be removed by passing 1–2 litres of mixed venous blood through a membrane lung optimised for CO_2 removal and that oxygenation could be achieved by mass flow of oxygen down the trachea during apnoea. This venovenous perfusion was subsequently combined with low frequency, pressure limited ventilation and used with great success by Gattinoni and others, who have obtained a survival rate of about 50% in very severe cases of ARDS.[52] The reduced blood flow results in less blood damage, and problems of bleeding have now been greatly reduced by percutaneous catheters and heparin bonded equipment. The technique requires expert medical and nursing care and can be carried out only in specialist centres. However, a recent randomised, controlled trial of the technique has not shown improved survival when compared with conventional methods of respiratory support.[53]

In recent years a third method of artificial gas exchange has been developed. This utilises a specially designed hollow fibre gas exchange device (the intravenous oxygenator or IVOX), which is inserted into the superior and inferior vena cavae. The fibres are permeable to gases but not to fluids and are flushed continuously with a stream of oxygen. The amount of gas exchanged across the membrane is not sufficient to provide full respiratory support, and its place in therapy has yet to be evaluated by clinical trials.[54]

Maintenance of the airway

The inability to secure and maintain an atraumatic, airtight connection with the trachea held back the development of intermittent positive pressure ventilation for several hundred years. This problem is still hindering the application of non-invasive methods of respiratory support.

In the experiments in which they showed the efficacy of artificial ventilation in open chest animals, Vesalius, Hooke, and Hunter used a tracheostomy to secure an airtight connection with the trachea. It was soon recognised that this was not practical for use in resuscitation, and in 1788 Charles Kite wrote an essay for the Royal Humane Society in which he described the use of both oral and nasal tubes for this purpose.[55] At the beginning of the 19th century P J Desault in France started to use oral intubation to relieve laryngeal obstruction in diphtheria,[56] and in 1858 John Snow described how he had anaesthetised a rabbit by inserting a wide bore tube into the trachea and connecting this to a bag containing chloroform.[57] F Trendelenburg, who was concerned with the problem of aspiration of blood during surgical operations on the upper air passages, modified this technique and in 1871 described how he had anaesthetised a patient by dropping chloroform onto a gauze covered funnel which was connected to a cuffed tracheostomy tube.[58] In 1880 William MacEwen first described the use of blind oral intubation in four patients, two of whom were intubated for over 24 hours.[56] In 1887 O'Dwyer, in New York, reported the use of prolonged oral intubation in the treatment of 50 patients with croup.[59] He initially used short tubes that were passed blindly into the larynx, but later he developed a longer tube that could be connected to a bellows to provide artificial ventilation.

The use of tracheal intubation in anaesthesia was pioneered by Fritz Kuhn in Germany, who described oral intubation with a flexible metal tube in 1901 and nasal intubation in 1902.[60] Kuhn was the first to describe the use of cocaine for topical anaesthesia of the larynx, and he passed the tubes blindly using a curved introducer. Direct laryngoscopy had been described by Kirstein in 1895,[61] but it was Elsberg (1912) and Chevalier Jackson (1913) who popularised the use of Jackson's laryngoscope for intubation.[60] In 1909 Meltzer and Auer described the insufflation technique of anaesthesia, in which the inhalational agent was delivered into the trachea through a narrow bore catheter, the expired gases exiting around the tube.[62] This technique remained popular until the mid-1920s, when the pioneer work of Magill and Rowbotham conclusively showed the advantages of tracheal intubation with a wide bore tube.[60] A cuffed endotracheal tube was first described by Dorrance in 1910 and reintroduced by Ralph Waters in 1928.[63] This greatly facilitated the use of controlled ventilation, a technique first used experimentally by Green and Janeway in 1910[14] and later used during ether anaesthesia by Guedel and Treweek[64] and advocated for thoracic surgery with cyclopropane anaesthesia by Waters in 1936.[65]

Endotracheal intubation was greatly facilitated by Griffith's introduction of curare in 1942,[66] but long term intubation was complicated by tissue reactions to the red rubber from which the tubes were made and by tracheal damage from the high pressure cuffs. Although it was hoped that the introduction of plastic tubes in the early 1950s would have abolished toxic reactions, they continued to occur. The trouble was traced to the plasticiser and has now been eliminated by subjecting all batches of plastic to implant testing. Tracheal damage from cuffs has now been reduced by the use of low pressure cuffs, but prolonged intubation and tracheostomy still result in an appreciable incidence of complications.

Non-invasive methods of respiratory support

Many patients with chronic respiratory or neuromuscular disease can maintain adequate ventilation for part or all of the day but need ventilatory assistance at night or during acute exacerbations of the chronic lung disease. In the past such patients were treated with fixed rate "negative" pressure devices, such as tank or cuirass ventilators; others were helped by the diaphragmatic movement generated by a rocking bed.

In recent years there has been increasing interest in the application of intermittent positive pressure ventilation by a closely fitting full face or nasal mask. The enormous improvement in the mechanics of patient triggering devices now enables such facilities to be incorporated into both cuirass and face mask ventilators, thereby greatly increasing patient acceptance. As a result, patients with chronic neuromuscular disease, or acute exacerbations of chronic obstructive lung disease, who would previously have been denied treatment, are now benefiting from intermittent periods of ventilatory assistance. The nocturnal application of continuous or intermittent positive pressure by nasal mask is also useful in treating patients with obstructive sleep apnoea.

Conclusions

Long term mechanical ventilation with intermittent positive pressure has now been practiced for over 40 years. Initially the technique was used to treat hypoventilation in patients who had relatively normal lungs but who were suffering from some abnormality of respiratory centre control or neuromuscular weakness. Providing that infection and technical complications were avoided, these patients created few problems.

As experience increased, mechanical ventilation was applied to the treatment of pulmonary complications after operation, pneumonia, severe asthma, acute-on-chronic lung disease, ARDS, and a wide range of other conditions. These patients often required high airway pressures to secure adequate alveolar ventilation, and pressures were often further increased by the need to apply positive end expiratory pressure to increase lung volume and so reduce the hypoxaemia resulting from alveolar collapse. The high airway pressures resulted in an increased incidence of barotrauma and a reduction in cardiac output, and this reduction often counteracted the beneficial effects of PEEP on oxygen delivery.

During the past 25 years the main thrust of research has been to develop techniques that minimise the harmful effects of mechanical ventilation. Unfortunately, many of these ventilatory modes can be generated only by sophisticated ventilators, which are not only more difficult to understand but also require more complex monitoring systems to ensure that they are functioning as intended.

Many machines are quite unnecessarily complex. There are two reasons for this state of affairs. Firstly, respiratory therapy in the United States is largely run by a group of highly intelligent and innovative technicians who have a close liaison with the manufacturers, who are selling in a very competitive market; this encourages the development of versatile machines with software that can be rapidly updated to keep up with the latest ventilatory mode. Secondly, when any new technique has been accepted into medical practice it becomes very difficult to persuade ethical committees that it should be submitted to a properly controlled trial. The difficulty of conducting such a trial in an intensive care unit is compounded by the relatively small numbers of patients available for study and by the heterogeneity of the patient population. Retrospective analyses have provided strong evidence that ventilators can reduce mortality in patients suffering from a primary ventilatory failure, but there is unfortunately little evidence to indicate that the use of any of the special ventilatory modes described above has had any further influence on mortality. Indeed the only two randomised, controlled studies on the use of PEEP suggest that its use is associated with an increase in mortality.[67, 68] I sincerely hope that one or more of my readers will eventually provide sound evidence that patient survival is improved by the application of one or more of the ventilatory modes discussed later in this book.

1 Vesalius A. *De humani corporis fabrica.* Basel, 1543.
2 Hooke R. An account of an experiment made by Mr Hook of preserving animals alive by blowing through their lungs with bellows. *Philosophical Transactions of the Royal Society* 1667;2:539–40.
3 Hunter J. Proposals for the recovery of people apparently drowned. *Philosophical Transactions of the Royal Society* 1776;66:412–25.
4 Leroy J. Recherches sur l'asphyxie. *J Physiol Expér Pathol* 1827;7:45–65, 1828;8:97–135.
5 Woollam CHM. The development of apparatus for intermittent negative pressure respiration. 1. 1832-1918. *Anaesthesia* 1976;31:537–47.
6 Woollam CHM. The development of apparatus for intermittent negative pressure respiration. 2. 1919–1976, with special reference to the development and uses of cuirass respirators. *Anaesthesia* 1976;31:666–85.
7 Fritsch PW. Experiences in the treatment by the barospirator. *Acta Med Scand* 1932;78:100–25.
8 Drinker P, Shaw LA. An apparatus for the prolonged administration of artificial respiration. 1. A design for adults and children. *J Clin Invest* 1929;7:229–47.
9 Bragg WH. The Bragg–Paul pulsator. *BMJ* 1938;ii:254.
10 Eve FC. Actuation of the inert diaphragm by a gravity method. *Lancet* 1932;ii:995–7.
11 Iron lungs. *Lancet* 1947;ii:193.
12 Macintosh RR. New use for the Both respirator. *Lancet* 1940;ii:745–6.

13 Kelleher WH. A new pattern of "iron lung" for the prevention and treatment of airway complications in paralytic disease. *Lancet* 1961;ii:1113–6.
14 Green NW, Janeway HH. Artificial respiration and intrathoracic oesophageal surgery. *Ann Surg* 1910;52:58–66.
15 Mushin WW, Rendell-Baker L, Thompson PW, Mapleson WW. *Automatic ventilation of the lungs*. 3rd ed. Oxford: Blackwell Scientific, 1980.
16 Jackson DE. A universal artificial respiration and closed anesthesia machine. *J Lab Clin Med* 1927;12:998–1002.
17 Mushin WW, Rendell-Baker L. *The principles of thoracic anaesthesia*. Oxford: Blackwell Scientific, 1953:598–661.
18 Frenckner P. Bronchial and tracheal catheterization and its clinical applicability. *Acta Otolaryngol (Stockh)* 1934;suppl 20:1–134.
19 Crafoord C. Pulmonary ventilation and anesthesia in major chest surgery. *J Thoracic Surg* 1940;9:237–53.
20 Moerch ET. Controlled respiration by means of special automatic machines as used in Sweden and Denmark. *Proc R Soc Med* 1947;40:603–7.
21 Rendell-Baker L, Pettis JL. The development of positive pressure ventilators. In: Atkinson RS, Boulton TB, eds. *The history of anaesthesia*. London: Royal Society of Medicine, 1989:402–25.
22 Wackers GL. Modern anesthesiological principles for bulbar polio: manual IPPR in the 1952 polio epidemic in Copenhagen. *Acta Anesthesiol Scand* 1994;38:420–31.
23 Lassen HCA, Bjorneboe M, Ibsen B, Neukirch F. Treatment of tetanus with curarisation, general anaesthesia, and intratracheal positive pressure ventilation. *Lancet* 1954;ii:1040–4.
24 Björk VO, Engström C-G. The treatment of ventilatory insufficiency after pulmonary resection with tracheostomy and prolonged artificial ventilation. *J Thorac Surg* 1955;30:356–67.
25 Mörch ET. History of mechanical ventilation. In: Kirby RR, Banner MJ, Downs JB, eds. *Clinical applications of ventilatory support*. Edinburgh: Churchill Livingstone, 1990:1–62.
26 Ashbaugh DG, Bigelow DB, Petty TL, Levine BE. Acute respiratory distress in adults. *Lancet* 1967;ii:319–23.
27 Kumar A, Falke KJ, Geffin B, Aldredge CF, Laver MB, Lowenstein E, et al. Continuous positive-pressure ventilation in acute respiratory failure. Effects on hemodynamics and lung function. *N Engl J Med* 1970;283:1430–6.
28 Sykes MK, Adams AP, Finlay WEI, McCormick PW, Economides A. The effects of end-expiratory inflation pressure on cardiorespiratory function in normo-, hypo-, and hypervolaemic dogs. *Br J Anaesth* 1970;42:669–77.
29 Qvist J, Pontoppidan H, Wilson RS, Lowenstein E, Laver MB. Hemodynamic responses to mechanical ventilation with PEEP: the effect of hypervolemia. *Anesthesiology* 1975;42:45–55.
30 Braunwald E, Binion JT, Morgan WL, Sarnoff SJ. Alterations in central blood volume and cardiac output induced by positive pressure breathing and counteracted by metaraminol (Aramine). *Circ Res* 1957;5:670–5.
31 Swan HJC, Ganz W, Forrester J, Marcus H, Diamond G, Chonette G. Cardiac catheterization with a flow-directed balloon tipped catheter. *N Engl J Med* 1970;283:447–50.
32 Sykes MK. Clinical measurement and clinical practice. *Anaesthesia* 1992;47:425–32.
33 Barach AL, Bickerman HA, Petty TL. Perspectives in pressure breathing. *Resp Care* 1975;20:627–42.
34 Gregory G, Kitterman J, Phibbs RH, Tooley WH, Hamilton WK. Continuous positive airway pressure with spontaneous respiration: a new method of increasing arterial oxygenation in the respiratory distress syndrome. *Pediatr Res* 1970;4:469–70.
35 Civetta JM, Brons R, Gabel JC. A simple and effective method of employing spontaneous positive pressure ventilation. Illustrative case reports. *J Thorac Cardiovasc Surg* 1972;63:312–17.
36 Kirby RR, Robison E, Schulz J, deLemos RA. Continuous flow ventilation as an alternative to assisted or controlled ventilation in infants. *Anesth Analg* 1972;51:871–5.
37 Downs JB, Klein EF, DeSautels D, Modell JH, Kirby RB. Intermittent mandatory ventilation: a new approach to weaning patients from mechanical ventilators. *Chest* 1973;64:331–5.

15

38 Hewlett AM, Platt AS, Terry VG. Mandatory minute volume: a new concept in weaning from mechanical ventilation. *Anaesthesia* 1977;**32**:163–9.
39 Brochard L. Inspiratory pressure support. *Eur J Anaesthesiol* 1993;**11**:29–36.
40 Jonzon A, Oberg PA, Sedin G, Sjöstrand U. High frequency positive pressure ventilation by endotracheal insufflation. *Acta Anaesthesiol Scand* 1971;suppl 43:1–43.
41 Carlon GC, Howland WS, Ray C, Miodownik S, Griffin JP, Groeger JS. High frequency jet ventilation. A prospective randomised evaluation. *Chest* 1983;**84**:551–9.
42 Hurst JM, Branson RD, Davis K, Barrette RR, Adams KS. Comparison of conventional mechanical ventilation and high-frequency ventilation. A prospective, randomized trial in patients with respiratory failure. *Ann Surg* 1990;**211**:486–91.
43 HIFI study group. High-frequency oscillatory ventilation compared with conventional mechanical ventilation in the treatment of respiratory failure in preterm infants. *N Engl J Med* 1989;**320**:88–93.
44 Bryan AC, Froese AB. Reflections on the HIFI trial. *Pediatrics* 1991;**87**:565–7.
45 Reynolds EOR. Effects of alterations in mechanical ventilator settings on pulmonary gas exchange in hyaline membrane disease. *Arch Dis Child* 1971;**46**:152–9.
46 Cole AGH, Weller SF, Sykes MK. Inverse ratio ventilation compared with PEEP in adult respiratory failure. *Intensive Care Med* 1984;**10**:227–32.
47 Stock MC, Downs JB, Frolicher DA. Airway pressure release ventilation. *Crit Care Med* 1987;**15**:462–6.
48 Hörmann Ch, Baum M, Putensen Ch, Mutz NJ, Benzer H. Biphasic positive airway pressure (BIPAP)—a new mode of ventilatory support. *Eur J Anaesthesiol* 1993;**11**:37–42.
49 Zapol WM, Snider MT, Hill DJ, Fallat RJ, Bartlett RH, Edmunds LH, *et al.* Extracorporeal membrane oxygenation in severe acute respiratory failure. A randomized prospective study. *JAMA* 1979;**242**:2193–6.
50 Pearson GA, Firmin RK, Sosnowski A. Review. Neonatal extracorporeal oxygenation. *Br J Hosp Med* 1992;**47**:646–53.
51 Kolobow T, Gattinoni L, Tomlinson T, Pierce JE. An alternative to breathing. *J Thorac Cardiovasc Surg* 1978;**75**:261–6.
52 Gattinoni L, Pesenti A, Marcolin R, Damia G. Extracorporeal support in acute respiratory failure. *Intensive Care World* 1988;**5**:42–45.
53 Morris AH, Wallace CJ, Menlove RL, Clemmer TP, Orme JF, Weaver LK, *et al.* Randomized clinical trial of pressure-controlled inverse ratio ventilation and extracorporeal CO_2 removal for adult respiratory distress syndrome. *Am J Respir Crit Care Med* 1994;**149**:295–305.
54 High KM, Snider MY, Richard R, Russell GB, Stene JK, Campbell DB, *et al.* Clinical trials of an intravenous oxygenator in patients with adult respiratory distress syndrome. *Anesthesiology* 1992;**77**:856–63.
55 Davison MHA. Endotracheal and other modern methods in the eighteenth century. *Br J Anaesth* 1951;**23**:238–45.
56 MacEwen W. Clinical observations on the introduction of tracheal tubes by the mouth instead of performing tracheotomy or laryngotomy. *BMJ* 1880;**2**:122–4, 163–5.
57 Snow J. *On chloroform and other anaesthetics.* London: Churchill, 1858:117.
58 Trendelenburg F. Tamponade der Trachea. *Arch Klin Chir* 1871;**12**:121–33.
59 O'Dwyer J. Fifty cases of croup in private practice treated by intubation of the larynx, with a description of the method and of the dangers incident thereto. *The Medical Record* 1887;**32**:557–61.
60 Gillespie NA. *Endotracheal anaesthesia.* 2nd ed. Madison: University of Wisconsin Press, 1948.
61 Hirsch NP, Smith GB, Hirsch PO. Alfred Kirstein. Pioneer of direct laryngoscopy. *Anaesthesia* 1986;**41**:42–5.
62 Meltzer SJ, Auer J. Continuous respiration without respiratory movements. *J Exp Med* 1909;**11**:622–5.
63 Waters RM, Rovenstine EA, Guedel AE. Endotracheal anesthesia and its historical development. *Anesth Analg* 1933;**12**:196–203.
64 Guedel AE, Treweek DN. Ether apnoeas. *Anesth Analg* 1934;**13**:263–4.
65 Waters RM. Carbon dioxide absorption from anaesthetic atmospheres. *Proc R Soc Med* 1936;**30**:11–22.

66 Griffith HR, Johnson GE. The use of curare in general anesthesia. *Anesthesiology* 1942;**3**:418–20.
67 Pepe PE, Hudson LD, Carrico CT. Early application of positive end-expiratory pressure in patients at risk for the adult respiratory distress syndrome. *N Engl J Med* 1984;**311**:281–6.
68 Carroll GC, Tuman KJ, Bransman B, Logas WG, Wool N, Goldin M, *et al*. Minimal positive end-expiratory pressure may be "best PEEP." *Chest* 1988;**93**:1020–5.

2 Physiological background to mechanical ventilation

There are two types of respiratory failure, which may occur separately or simultaneously: ventilatory failure and hypoxaemic failure. Ventilatory failure may be caused by a decrease in central respiratory drive, neuromuscular weakness, or an increase in the impedances to respiration. In this type of failure the alveolar ventilation is inadequate to clear the CO_2 production so that there is an increase in alveolar and arterial PCO_2, and a decrease in alveolar and arterial PO_2 when the patient is breathing air (fig 2.1). Although

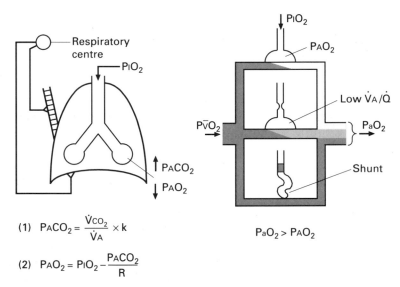

(1) $\quad PACO_2 = \dfrac{\dot{V}CO_2}{\dot{V}A} \times k$

(2) $\quad PAO_2 = PIO_2 - \dfrac{PACO_2}{R}$

$PaO_2 > PAO_2$

Fig 2.1 The two types of respiratory failure. (left): Ventilatory failure. Equation 1 shows that alveolar PCO_2 ($PACO_2$) increases because alveolar ventilation ($\dot{V}A$) is insufficient to eliminate CO_2 production ($\dot{V}CO_2$). The simplified alveolar gas equation (2) shows that increase in $PACO_2$ results in decrease in alveolar PO_2 (PAO_2). PAO_2 can be returned to normal levels by increasing inspired oxygen (PIO_2); k is a constant to correct for units of measurement; R is respiratory exchange ratio, normally 0.8. (right): Hypoxaemic failure. Arterial PO_2 (PaO_2) is less than PAO_2 (calculated from the alveolar gas equation) because of venous admixture from ventilation-perfusion inequalities ($\dot{V}A/\dot{Q}$) and from right-to-left shunt. Both types of failure may occur in the same patient.

Types of respiratory failure

Ventilatory

- Causes
  Decrease in central respiratory drive
  Neuromuscular weakness
  Increased impedance to ventilation

- Results
  Alveolar and arterial PCO_2 increase
  Alveolar and arterial PO_2 decrease when patient is breathing air
  Hypoxaemia relieved by breathing 30–35% oxygen

Hypoxaemic

- Causes
  Ventilation-perfusion inequalities
  Increase in intrapulmonary shunt (atelectasis, consolidation, pulmonary oedema)

- Results
  Alveolar and arterial PCO_2 normal or decreased
  Alveolar PO_2 normal or increased; arterial PO_2 decreased
  Increased inspired oxygen concentration:
    Reduces hypoxaemia due to ventilation-perfusion inequalities
    Has little effect on hypoxaemia due to shunt

the hypoxaemia can be relieved by breathing oxygen, this is only a temporary expedient; some form of ventilatory assistance is usually needed to restore ventilation to normal levels.

The second form of respiratory failure, the hypoxaemic type, is due to ventilation–perfusion inequalities or to an increase in intrapulmonary shunt. The latter is most commonly caused by atelectasis, consolidation, or oedema. Hypoxaemic failure results in a decrease in arterial PO_2 with no increase in alveolar or arterial PCO_2. Indeed, reflex stimulation from the lungs or peripheral chemoreceptors may cause arterial PCO_2 to be less than normal. Hypoxaemia due to ventilation–perfusion inequalities can be abolished by increasing the inspired oxygen concentration to 30–35%, but giving oxygen has a much smaller effect on arterial PO_2 when the hypoxaemia is due to shunt, since the shunted blood cannot take part in gas exchange. Treatment must, therefore, be directed towards re-expansion of collapsed areas of lung.

Subsequent chapters deal in more detail with the pathophysiology of respiratory failure and with methods of respiratory support designed to augment alveolar ventilation or to re-expand collapsed areas of lung. Since all these techniques have physiological implications, it is first necessary to consider how they may affect normal physiology.

19

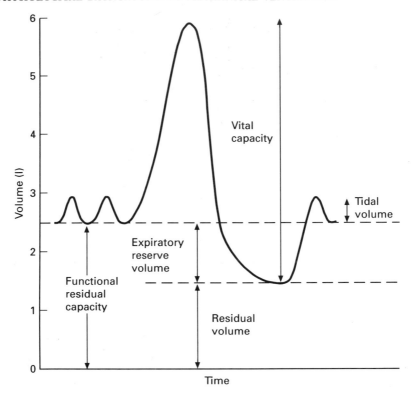

Fig 2.2 The lung volumes. The subject breathed normally and then took a maximal inspiration and expiration. Supine posture and abdominal distension reduce the expiratory reserve volume. The residual volume increases with age and with airways obstruction.

Respiratory mechanics

Resting end expiratory position

The first factor to consider in any discussion of respiratory mechanics is the resting position of the lung-chest wall combination. This is normally defined by the volume of gas contained in the lung – the functional residual capacity (fig 2.2). The resting position is determined by the opposing forces generated by the elastic recoil of the lung and the outward recoil of the chest wall. The chest wall is pulled inwards by the lung and so is about 1 litre below its own natural resting position (fig 2.3). The pressure gradient generated by the elastic recoil of the lung depends on the lung's elasticity and on the lung volume. The opposing pressure gradient developed by the chest wall is also volume dependent but is, in addition, affected by body position and gravity.

In the upright position the abdominal contents exert little upward pressure on the diaphragm, but when the guts are distended or the patient is placed in

20

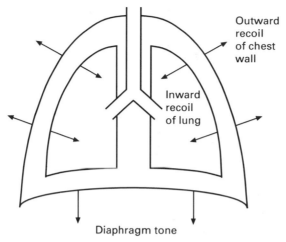

Outward
recoil
of chest
wall

Inward
recoil
of lung

Diaphragm tone

Fig 2.3 The opposing forces governing the resting end expiratory position (functional residual capacity).

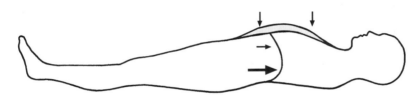

Fig 2.4 Forces tending to reduce functional residual capacity. Hydrostatic pressure exerted by abdominal contents is maximal in dependent zones and is increased by ascites or intestinal distension. Obesity increases intra-abdominal pressure and may also impair rib movement.

the supine or head down position the pressure exerted by the abdominal contents forces the diaphragm up into the chest, so reducing the functional residual capacity (fig 2.4). Since the abdominal contents behave as a liquid, the hydrostatic pressure is greatest in the dependent areas. This tends to distort the shape of the diaphragm, so that the dependent parts of the diaphragm move further up into the chest than the non-dependent parts. When the subject breathes spontaneously the hydrostatic pressure effects are opposed by the greater mechanical efficiency resulting from the increased convexity of the dependent parts of the diaphragm and by an increase in diaphragm tone, but when the diaphragm is paralysed the hydrostatic pressure is transmitted directly to the underlying lung.

These gravitationally induced changes may reduce the FRC from the normal upright value of 2.5–3.0 l to a volume of 1.5–2.0 l in the supine, paralysed patient, a volume close to the normal residual volume (figs 2.2 and 2.5). This naturally predisposes to alveolar collapse in dependent zones of the

21

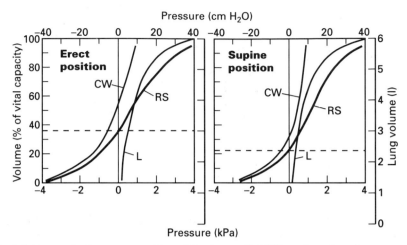

Fig 2.5 Pressure/volume curves of lung (L), chest wall (CW), and total respiratory system (RS) show how change in shape of the chest wall curve resulting from adopting supine position leads to decrease in functional residual capacity (dotted line). The lung volume scale (right) shows that the residual volume (volume of gas remaining in the lung after a maximal expiration, normally about 1.3 l or 20% of total lung capacity) is not included.

lung and this, in turn, produces a further reduction in FRC. Obesity augments the reduction in FRC in the supine position because obesity increases the hydrostatic pressure in the abdomen, while the extra weight on the chest wall reduces the volume of the thoracic cage. Gut distension or ascites will also tend to splint the diaphragm. The reduction in FRC can be reversed by the application of a positive end expiratory pressure (PEEP) to the trachea, but this will tend to expand alveoli in the more compliant non-dependent zones of the lung, as re-expansion of collapsed areas in dependent zones occurs only at much higher levels of PEEP.

Impedances to ventilation

There are three impedances to ventilation – the elastic recoil of the lungs and chest wall; the frictional resistance to gas flow in the airways; and the viscous resistance resulting from the deformation of the tissues. The last is relatively small and can usually be ignored. At normal breathing frequencies the pressure required to inflate the lungs may thus be considered to have two components – that required to drive the inspired gas along the airways and that required to inflate the alveoli (fig 2.6). However, during high frequency ventilation it is also necessary to consider the force required to accelerate the mass of the lung and chest wall (the inertance).

The lungs and chest wall. The elastic recoil of the lung is generated by the elasticity of the lung tissue and by the surface tension of the fluid lining the

22

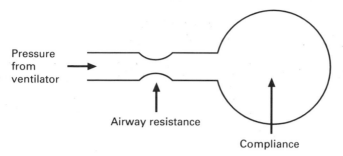

Fig 2.6 The major impedances to ventilation are airway resistance and total thoracic compliance.

alveoli. Normally the surface tension forces are minimised by the presence of surfactant, a complex lipoprotein secreted by the type 2 cells in the alveoli. In normal lungs about 50% of the recoil pressure is due to surface tension forces, but the proportion is greatly increased when surfactant is deficient. As shown in figure 2.5, the pressure-volume curves of the lung and chest wall are approximately linear in the tidal volume range, so that their elastic properties can be defined by the compliance – the volume change per unit pressure. In a normal, supine 70 kg adult the compliances of the lungs and chest wall are similar and approximately equal to 1 l kPa^{-1} (100 ml/cm H$_2$O). To achieve a volume change of, say, 0.1 l it is necessary to apply a pressure difference of 0.1 kPa (1 cm H$_2$O) across the lung and 0.1 kPa (1 cm H$_2$O) across the chest

---

Impedances to ventilation

Elastic recoil of lungs and chest wall
- Recoil pressure reduced in emphysema: compliance and FRC increased
- Tissue distensibility decreased in fibrosis: compliance and FRC decreased
- In acute lung disease reduced compliance is mainly due to decreased volume of ventilated lung

Frictional resistance to gas flow
- Resistance is non-linear and higher in expiration than inspiration
- Increased by presence of tracheal or tracheostomy tube and secretions
- Increased in asthma, chronic obstructive airways disease, and pulmonary oedema
- Increased resistance results in slower filling and emptying of lungs, and intrinsic PEEP; the latter increases mean intrathoracic pressure, so decreasing cardiac output and increasing airway pressure needed to start inspiration

Viscous resistance of tissues
- Relatively constant and small proportion of total work of breathing

---

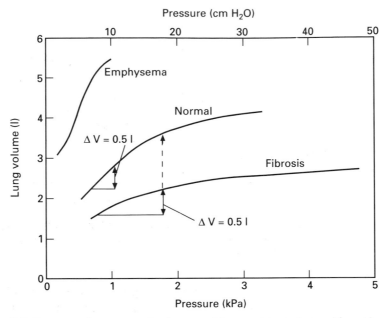

Fig 2.7 Pressure-volume curves in the normal lung and in patients with emphysema or fibrosis. Delivery of 500 ml tidal volume into a lung with reduced compliance (due to fibrosis, for example) will result in a high airway pressure, which may overdistend alveoli in normal areas of lung.

wall. Thus the compliance of the lung-chest wall combination is $0.1/(0.1 + 0.1) = 0.5$ l kPa^{-1} (50 ml/cm H$_2$O) and an inflation pressure of 2 kPa (20 cm H$_2$O) is required to increase the lung volume by 1 litre.

In patients with normal lungs there is little variation in the elasticity of the lung tissue, so that differences in compliance between individuals are mainly due to differences in lung volume. This variability may be eliminated by expressing the values in terms of the "specific compliance," the compliance divided by the lung volume at which the measurement is made (usually the FRC). This is normally about 0.05 in the upright position.

The lungs of patients with emphysema contain fewer elastic fibres than normal, so that the recoil pressure at any given lung volume is reduced. This results in an increase in compliance and in FRC. Fibrosis decreases the distensibility of the lung tissue, so that compliance and FRC are reduced (fig 2.7). In patients with acute lung disease such as pulmonary oedema, consolidation, or collapse, however, the reduction in compliance is due mainly to a reduction in the volume of ventilated lung and not to changes in the elasticity of the remaining lung tissue. In such circumstances the delivery of a normal tidal volume may result in high alveolar pressures, which may cause overdistension and damage in the relatively normal, ventilated areas of lung. This seems to be a common cause of barotrauma (see chapter 5).

24

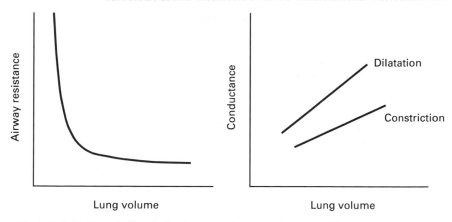

Fig 2.8 (left) Hyperbolic relation between airway resistance and lung volume. (right) If conductance (the reciprocal of resistance) is plotted against lung volume, a straight line results. This facilitates comparisons of airway calibre.

The airways. The airways are normally held open by the elastic recoil of the adjacent lung tissue, and this in turn depends on the "negative" (subatmospheric) pressure in the pleural space. The airways therefore expand and contract in parallel with the lungs, though at any given lung volume their diameter is greater during inspiration than during expiration since the absolute pleural pressure* is lower during inspiration than expiration. Since the resistance to laminar flow of gas through the airways is inversely related to the fourth power of the radius of the airways, airway resistance increases with decreasing lung volume. The relationship is approximately hyperbolic, with a considerable increase in resistance at low lung volumes (fig 2.8). If the relation is expressed as conductance (the reciprocal of resistance) against lung volume, it becomes a straight line. The slope of this line, which is independent of lung volume, is specific conductance. This provides a useful measure of the effect of bronchoactive drugs on the airways.

Although it would be expected that most airway resistance would be situated in the narrower airways in the periphery of the lung, the narrower airways actually contribute less than one quarter of the total pressure drop between mouth and alveoli because the velocity of airflow is greatly reduced by the large increase in total cross sectional area resulting from the repeated

---

* The terms "negative" or "subatmospheric" pressure are frequently used in the literature concerned with mechanical ventilation. However, confusion can arise in descriptions of a change in the numerical value of a "negative" pressure. I will use the traditional term "negative pressure" (hereafter without inverted commas) to describe ventilation by the application of a subatmospheric pressure around the chest but not to describe changes in pleural pressure. To avoid confusion these will be related to the absolute scale of pressure in which zero is the pressure in a complete vacuum and atmospheric pressure is 760 mm Hg, 101.325 kPa, or 1013 mbar.

branching of the airways. The major pressure drop therefore occurs at the level of the segmental bronchi. The airway resistance in the normal subject is 0.1–0.2 kPa l^{-1} s (1–2 cm $H_2O/l/s$).

Airway resistance is increased in patients with chronic obstructive airways disease and may exceed 2–3 kPa l^{-1} s (20–30 cm $H_2O/l/s$) in patients with asthma. The mechanisms causing the increase in airway resistance are complex and include increased bronchial muscle tone, mucosal oedema, the presence of secretions, and the loss of elastic recoil within the lung. Patients with increased airway resistance often have hyperinflated lungs and this may decrease the efficiency of the diaphragm and other respiratory muscles. The degree of hyperinflation is often increased by dynamic compression of the larger airways resulting from an increase in pleural pressure secondary to expiratory muscle activity. This may limit peak expiratory flow.[1]

The presence of a tracheal or tracheostomy tube also increases airway resistance, a total resistance of 0.5–1.0 kPa l^{-1} s (5–10 cm $H_2O/l/sec$) being commonly encountered in adults intubated with an 8 mm or 9 mm tracheal tube.[2] It is difficult to specify the resistance accurately as turbulent flow makes it non-linear, resistance increasing with flow rate. The resistance is also affected by the geometry of the tube and connections, and is increased by the presence of even a thin film of secretions on the inner wall of the tube.[3]

This high resistance has two important consequences. Firstly, while gas is flowing to and from the patient the pressure recorded in the ventilator tubing will be different from the pressure existing in the alveoli. Since expiratory resistance is greater than inspiratory resistance (because of the higher absolute pleural pressure during expiration), the measurement of mean airway pressure may not reflect mean alveolar pressure. Secondly, the tube resistance will augment the effects of any pre-existing increase in airway resistance and so will delay the emptying of the alveoli during the expiratory phase. If the total resistance is increased to such an extent that expiratory flow is still continuing when the machine cycles to inspiration, the alveolar pressure will never fall to atmospheric, thus producing the so called auto, alveolar, or intrinsic PEEP (fig 2.9). An intrinsic PEEP may be detected by occluding the airway at the end of the expiration and measuring the equilibrium airway pressure after 3 or 4 seconds.[4] A pause button, which automatically occludes both inspiratory and expiratory valves, is now provided on many ventilators to facilitate this measurement.

Intrinsic PEEP has two major effects. Firstly, there is an increase in alveolar and intrathoracic pressure throughout the respiratory cycle. This tends to decrease cardiac output and also increases the pressures measured by central venous or pulmonary artery catheters. The second major consequence of intrinsic PEEP is that the airway pressure required to initiate inspiration is increased (fig 2.9). The spontaneously breathing patient must develop a subatmospheric intrathoracic pressure equal to the alveolar pressure before inspiration can start.[5] This obviously increases the work of breathing and also

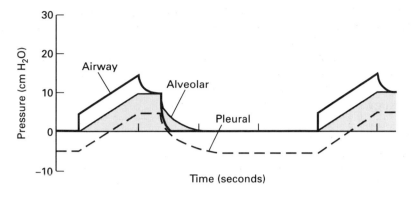

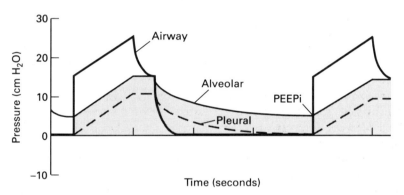

Fig 2.9 Generation of intrinsic PEEP (PEEPi). (top) Airway, alveolar, and pleural pressures during controlled ventilation with end inspiratory pause in patient with normal airway resistance. Note that the lung empties quickly so that alveolar pressure (shaded) equals atmospheric pressure at end of expiration. (bottom) Changes resulting from doubling of resistance. Alveolar pressure is higher than airway pressure at end of expiration, so generating PEEPi. At beginning of inspiration, airway pressure must exceed PEEPi before airflow will occur. The increase in mean alveolar pressure will result in an increase in mean pleural pressure, which will tend to decrease cardiac output.

delays the triggering of an assisted breath. During controlled ventilation with a constant inspiratory flow, intrinsic PEEP causes the increase in airway pressure at the start of inspiration to exceed the decrease in pressure at the onset of the end inspiratory pause.

Increases in airway resistance may occur in other conditions such as pulmonary oedema and the adult respiratory distress syndrome. It was originally thought that this increase was associated with the decrease in lung volume in these conditions, but recent studies, which show that the resistance increases with increasing PEEP, suggest that it is probably related

27

to stress adaptation phenomena or to time constant inhomogeneities.[6] Measurements of lung mechanics in patients with ARDS requiring an applied PEEP of, say, 10 cm H_2O show that total thoracic compliance may be reduced to 0.3–0.5 l kPa^{-1} (30–50 ml/cm H_2O), total airway resistance may be 0.8–1.2 kPa l^{-1} s (8–12 cm $H_2O/l/s$), and intrinsic PEEP may be 5–10 cm H_2O.[7]

Time constants and dynamic compliance

When the lungs are exposed to a constant airway pressure for an infinite time they will fill to a volume that is determined by the applied pressure and the total thoracic compliance, a high airway pressure or a high compliance resulting in a larger tidal volume. However, the instantaneous flow rate during the period of filling will depend not only on the difference in pressure between the alveoli and the source of pressure, but also on the airway resistance.

With a constant pressure source, the pressure difference is maximal at the beginning of inspiration when alveolar pressure is zero and then falls exponentially, final equilibrium between the applied pressure and alveolar pressure occurring theoretically only in infinite time (fig 2.10). The exponential decrease in flow rate during inspiration results in an exponential increase in volume of the lung. It is a characteristic of an exponential pattern of change that the rate of change can be predicted from the time constant, 63% of the change being completed in one time constant, 87% in two time constants, 95% in three, and 99% in four. In the lung the time constant (T) can be calculated from the total thoracic compliance (C) and the airway resistance (R):

$$T \text{ (secs)} = C \text{ (l kPa}^{-1}) \times R \text{ (kPa l}^{-1} \text{ s)}$$

$$\text{or } T \text{ (secs)} = C \text{ (l/cm } H_2O) \times R \text{ (cm } H_2O/l/s)$$

For a normal lung the time constant will be 1 l $kPa^{-1} \times 0.2$ kPa l^{-1} s $= 0.2$ seconds, so the alveoli will be filled to 99% of the final volume (which they would achieve if infinite time were allowed) after 0.8 seconds. It can be seen that the time constant will increase if airway resistance is increased (which would tend to decrease the inspiratory flow rate), or if compliance is increased (which would increase the volume that has to enter the lungs to generate a pressure equal to the applied pressure). Conversely, a low airway resistance or a stiff lung will shorten the time required to achieve pressure equilibrium between the mouth and the alveoli.

As changes in compliance or resistance affect the rate of filling of the lungs in response to a constant applied pressure, they may be expected to influence the tidal volume delivered by a ventilator if the duration of inspiration is limited (fig 2.10). In the normal lung the time constants of the individual

28

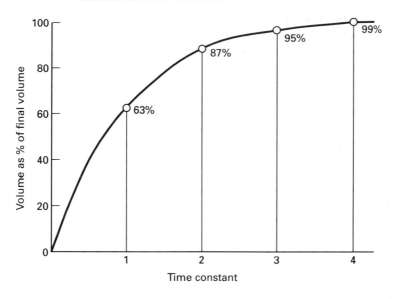

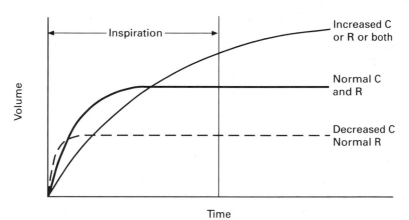

Fig 2.10 (top) Pattern of exponential filling of the lung in response to application of constant pressure at the mouth. (bottom) Effect of changes of compliance (C) and resistance (R). With an infinite duration of inspiration the volume delivered depends only on airway pressure and compliance. However, an increased C or R increases the time taken to reach pressure equilibrium between ventilator and alveoli, so tidal volume may be decreased if duration of inspiration is limited.

alveolar units seem to be short enough to ensure that the end inspiratory pressure in most of the alveoli reaches equilibrium with the applied pressure during the normal period of inspiration. Indeed, this seems to be the case

29

even at frequencies as high as 50–60 bpm in patients with normal lungs, for measurements of dynamic compliance (calculated from measurements made at the normal or higher breathing frequency) approximate to measurements of static compliance (made during a breathhold).

In patients with lung disease there is often a wide variation in time constants throughout the lung, so that some alveoli do not fill in the time available. This causes the dynamic compliance to be less than the static value, and may result in ventilation-perfusion inequalities. Prolonging inspiration in the technique of inverse ratio ventilation may decrease these inequalities by providing adequate time for all the alveolar units to attain equilibrium with the applied pressure, but it may introduce other problems due to incomplete emptying of alveoli with long time constants (see chapter 5).

During expiration it is the alveolar pressure that drives the gas through the airways; once again, air flow is maximal at the beginning of expiration, when the difference between alveolar pressure and ambient pressure is maximal, and then decreases in an approximately exponential manner. (The deviation from a true exponential in both phases of respiration is caused by changes in airway resistance with lung volume.)

In some ventilators the pressure generated at the mouth varies during inspiration. In others the ventilator generates a pattern of flow rather than pressure. Under such circumstances the above analysis will not be applicable to the inspiratory phase, though the exponential decline in flow during expiration remains unchanged. However, time constant inequalities are a potent source of ventilation-perfusion inequalities, and their effects may generally be ameliorated by prolonging the duration of inspiration and expiration. Unfortunately, there may be little scope for using this manoeuvre, because the resulting decrease in respiratory frequency may produce an unacceptable reduction in alveolar ventilation.

Measurement of compliance and resistance

The standard method of measuring compliance is to measure the volume change resulting from a given change in inflation pressure.[8] During spontaneous ventilation the patient generates a number of breathholds at different lung volumes and the volume change is measured by a spirometer, but in the apnoeic patient the volume change is usually generated by injecting an oxygen enriched gas from a large, calibrated syringe. Ideally, pressure measurements are made at several different lung volumes so that a pressure-volume curve can be plotted. To determine lung compliance it is necessary to measure the difference in pressure between the alveoli and pleural space, while chest wall compliance is derived by measuring the difference in pressure between the pleural space and the atmosphere (fig 2.11). Pleural pressure can be measured directly if pleural drains are present but is usually obtained by measuring the pressure within a thin walled balloon inserted into

Measurements of compliance and resistance

Compliance
- Static: change in volume related to change in pressure during zero flow period of 2–3 seconds
- Dynamic: change in volume related to change in compliance component of pressure during ventilation at normal respiratory frequencies
- Dynamic compliance<static compliance when time constants increased

Resistance
- Pressure difference between mouth and alveoli related to flow rate

Normal values
- Total thoracic compliance: 1.0 l kPa^{-1} (erect); 0.5–0.75 l kPa^{-1} (supine)
- Airway resistance: 0.1–0.2 kPa l^{-1} s; 0.5–1.0 kPa l^{-1} s (intubated)

the oesophagus. However, care is necessary to ensure that the measurement is not affected by the weight of the heart when the patient is in the supine position. Oesophageal contractions may also downgrade the accuracy of the measurement.

The appropriate pressure difference for the measurement of total thoracic compliance is from the alveoli to atmosphere. It is difficult to measure total thoracic compliance in spontaneously breathing patients, as they have to learn to relax the respiratory muscles at a series of lung volumes while

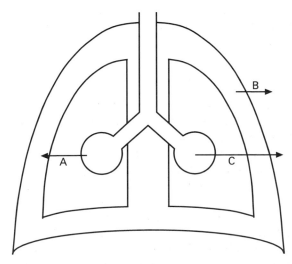

Fig 2.11 Pressure differences measured to determine compliance. A = lung compliance, B = chest wall compliance, C = total thoracic compliance. Pleural pressure is usually derived from measurements of oesophageal pressure.

31

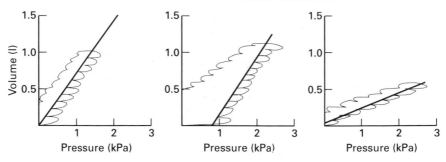

Fig 2.12 Pressure-volume curves recorded by injecting 100 ml aliquots of oxygen into the lungs from a large syringe. Each aliquot results in a rise in pressure, which settles at a new level in 2–3 seconds. The compliance curve is plotted by joining these plateaus of pressure where flow is zero. The hysteresis between the inflation curve (right) and deflation curve (left) is due to gas exchange during measurement. (left) Normal lungs; (centre) early ARDS – inflection point on inspiratory curve may be caused by recruitment of collapsed alveoli or presence of intrinsic PEEP; (right) late (fibrotic) stage of ARDS.

pressure and volume measurements are made. However, there is little difficulty in measuring the inflation pressure and expired volume when ventilation is controlled by a positive or negative pressure ventilator. As the measurement of pleural pressure in the supine position is subject to error, whereas the measurement of the total pressure difference across the lungs and chest wall is easy, most clinicians use the measurement of total thoracic compliance as an index of the mechanical condition of the lung in the paralysed patient. However, it must be remembered that changes in posture and abdominal distension may change chest wall compliance and so affect the measurement.

The simplest method of measuring lung, chest wall, or total thoracic compliance in the paralysed patient is to ventilate the lungs with a high concentration of oxygen (to ensure that the patient does not become hypoxic during the measurement), and then to disconnect the patient from the ventilator and inject 200–300 ml aliquots of oxygen into the lungs from a large syringe while the appropriate pressure difference is measured.[9] Each increment of volume is followed by a 2–3 second pause so that a line can be drawn through the points of zero flow and pressure equilibrium to define the pressure-volume curve. Alternatively, the curve may be established by providing a continuous, slow (1–5 l/min) inflation which minimises the pressure drop down the airways due to airway resistance.[10] As may be seen in fig 2.12, there is noticeable hysteresis between the inflation and deflation slopes, which is due to continuing gas exchange during the measurement.[11] This obviously leads to an error in the slopes of both the inspiratory and expiratory limbs.

In patients in the early stages of pulmonary oedema or ARDS there is often an inflection in the inspiratory limb, which is believed to mark the pressure at

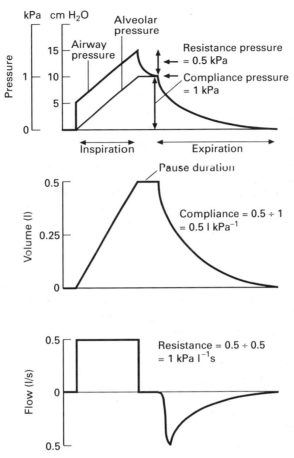

Fig 2.13 On line measurement of dynamic compliance and airway resistance using a constant flow ventilator with end inspiratory pause. Compliance is calculated by dividing tidal volume by compliance pressure, and resistance is calculated by dividing resistance pressure drop by flow rate.

which collapsed alveoli begin to re-expand. This point has been used as a guide to the required level of PEEP.[9, 12, 13] In patients with an increased airway resistance, however, it can also be due to the presence of intrinsic PEEP.[14] In early ARDS the slope of the ascending limb of the curve above this point, which defines the specific compliance of the expanded areas of lung, is still normal. In the later stages of the disease the inflection point tends to disappear and the slope of the ascending limb becomes more horizontal (fig 2.12). This reduction in specific compliance is believed to correspond to the development of fibrotic changes in the lung.

A number of ventilators are equipped with monitoring systems that enable compliance and resistance to be calculated on line. The principle is illustrated

33

in fig 2.13. The ventilator is set to deliver inspired gas at a constant flow. When flow starts there is a step increase in pressure at the ventilator end of the tracheal tube due to the presence of the airflow resistance. If the flow rate is 0.5 ls^{-1} and the resistance is 1 kPa l^{-1} s (10 cm $H_2O/l/sec$) the pressure drop along the airways will be 0.5 kPa (5 cm H_2O). However, an additional pressure is required to distend the alveoli. As compliance is assumed to be linear, and flow rate is constant, this pressure will also increase linearly and will be added to the airway resistance pressure. If the tidal volume is 0.5 l and compliance 0.5 l kPa^{-1} (50 ml/cm H_2O), there will be a pressure in the alveoli of 1 kPa (10 cm H_2O) at the end of inspiration.

While flow continues it is not possible to tell how much of the pressure at the mouth is due to resistance and how much to total thoracic compliance. However, if an end inspiratory pause is introduced, the flow resistance component will disappear and the remaining pressure will be due to the elastic recoil of the lungs and chest wall. Compliance may then be calculated by relating the plateau pressure to the expired volume, and resistance can be calculated by relating the step change in pressure at the beginning or end of inspiration to the measured flow rate. Because airway resistance decreases as the lungs are inflated there is a small difference between the two step changes; it is customary to use the pressure drop at the start of the pause for calculating resistance since the increase at the beginning of inspiration may be influenced by the presence of intrinsic PEEP (fig 2.9). It is, of course, essential to ensure that the duration of the plateau is long enough to ensure that equilibrium is reached between the airway pressure and the pressure in the alveoli (a minimum of 0.2 seconds). Although there are a number of absolute errors in the measurements associated with the design of each ventilator, there is a good enough correlation between true and measured values for the computerised results to be used as an indication of trends.[15]

This type of analysis can be applied to any ventilator waveform, though the separation of the resistance and compliance components of the airway pressure trace is more complicated (fig 2.14). When the flow pattern is known, changes in shape of the resultant pressure pattern can yield an early warning of changes in resistance and compliance. These may be of great therapeutic importance. Some examples of the effects of changes of compliance and resistance on pressure, flow and volume traces are shown in the next chapter (figs 3.2 and 3.3).

Other automated methods of measuring compliance have recently been introduced. In one of these the airway is occluded for 5 second periods at randomly chosen lung volumes during inspiration and expiration and the resulting pressure and volume points are plotted automatically by the computer.[16] This method completely abolishes the hysteresis due to gas exchange and generates very reproducible results. The intercept of these pressure-volume curves with the pressure axis also provides an accurate method of measuring intrinsic PEEP.[17]

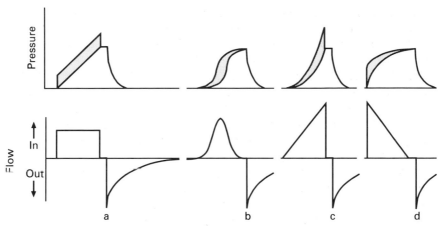

Fig 2.14 Airway pressure waveforms with common inspiratory flow patterns. Shading indicates airway resistance component of airway pressure, which parallels flow rate. As compliance is unchanged, the pattern of volume change during inspiration and expiration is shown by lines bounding clear area on pressure trace. Peak airway pressure is maximal with ascending ramp (c) and least with descending flow waveform (d). However, mean pressure is greatest with descending flow waveform (d), least with ascending waveform (c), and intermediate with constant (a) and sine wave (b) waveforms. Note that the expiratory flow trace has been truncated in (b), (c), and (d).

Ventilatory requirements

The total ventilation required to maintain a normal arterial PCO_2 depends on the CO_2 production ($\dot{V}CO_2$) and on the effective alveolar ventilation ($\dot{V}A$):

$$PaCO_2 = \frac{\dot{V}CO_2}{\dot{V}A} \times k$$

where k is a factor which corrects for the units of measurement. $\dot{V}CO_2$ is normally expressed in ml/min STPD (standard temperature and pressure, dry) whereas $\dot{V}A$ is expressed in l/min BTPS (body temperature and pressure, saturated). When $PaCO_2$ is expressed in mm Hg, $k = 0.863$, and when it is expressed in kPa, $k = 0.115$. The relation between ventilation and PCO_2 is hyperbolic (fig 2.15). Hyperventilation reduces the concentration of CO_2 in the alveolar gas and this, together with the dead space, prevents arterial PCO_2 values decreasing below 1.5–2.0 kPa. When ventilatory failure occurs there is a progressive retention of CO_2, which results in an increase in body stores. However, when a new equilibrium has been reached the higher alveolar CO_2 level once again enables the whole of the body's CO_2 production to be excreted with the reduced alveolar ventilation.

The CO_2 production depends on body size, age, and sex and is approximately 200 ml/min at rest. It increases by about 7% for each rise in body temperature of 1°C and also increases when the respiratory exchange ratio is

35

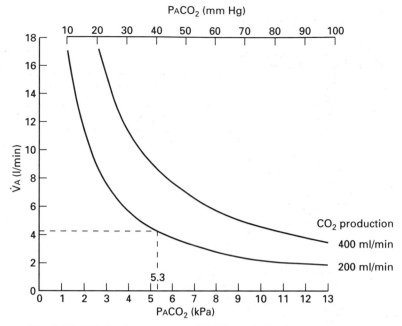

Fig 2.15 Relation between arterial PCO$_2$ and alveolar minute volume.

increased by a switch to carbohydrate metabolism.[18] Under such conditions large volumes of ventilation may be required to clear the CO_2 load; this may seriously impede weaning from a ventilator.

The effective alveolar minute ventilation ($\dot{V}A$) depends on the frequency (f), the exhaled tidal volume (VE), and on the apparatus dead space (VD^{App}) and physiological dead space (VD^P):

$$\dot{V}A = (V_E \times f) - [(V_D{}^{App} + V_D{}^P) \times f]$$

The apparatus dead space is usually considered to be the volume of the connections and other devices situated between the patient Y piece and the tracheal tube (fig 2.16). However, any inefficiency in CO_2 elimination resulting from rebreathing in any part of the breathing system will have the same effects on CO_2 elimination as adding an extra dead space, so the degree of rebreathing is often quantified by equating it with an equivalent volume of apparatus dead space. Rebreathing may occur if the flow of fresh gas into a T piece system is inadequate, or if one way inspiratory or expiratory valves are incompetent. In the early years of mechanical ventilation it was often necessary to increase tidal volume to facilitate patient synchronisation with the ventilator. An artificial dead space was then added to the breathing system to restore arterial PCO$_2$ towards normal levels.

The physiological dead space is normally about 150 ml or a third of the

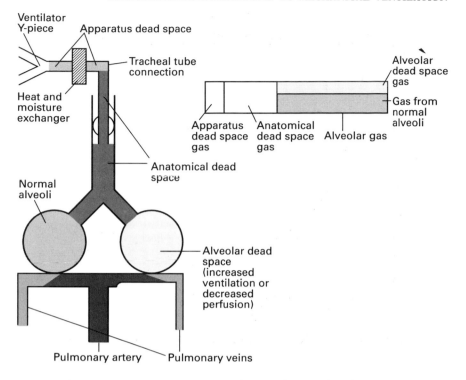

Fig 2.16 (above) Components of dead space; (below) components of expired gas. Gas from the apparatus and anatomical dead space (containing no CO_2) is expired first, and followed by alveolar gas. The latter is a mixture of gas from normally ventilated and perfused alveoli and gas from alveoli with a high ventilation/perfusion ratio. Since the CO_2 concentration in the latter is lower than in normal alveoli, unit volume of ventilation removes less CO_2 than it would if delivered to normal alveoli. This source of inefficiency is equated with an imaginary dead space at alveolar level. It also causes end-tidal PCO_2 to be lower than arterial PCO_2. (See also Fig 7.1, p. 156.)

tidal volume. It depends on the anatomical dead space (the volume of the conducting airways) and on the alveolar dead space (which is a measure used to quantify the inefficiency of gas exchange at alveolar level). The anatomical dead space is normally about 2 ml/kg body weight, but the pharyngeal component may vary by 40 ml with extrusion or retraction of the jaw. The tracheal component increases by about 30 ml for each litre increase in lung volume and also increases in old age. Atropine and bronchodilator drugs may increase anatomical dead space by up to 50%. The low flow rates associated with tidal volumes below about 200 ml result in the stasis of gas around the periphery of the major airways so that the effective anatomical dead space becomes less than the internal volume of the airways. Cardiac pulsations may also assist gas mixing in the airways. These mechanisms helps to maintain

37

CO_2 excretion during hypoventilation and so complement the increased CO_2 elimination per unit alveolar ventilation resulting from the increased level of alveolar CO_2.

In a lung with perfect matching of ventilation and perfusion there would be no alveolar dead space. In patients with normal lungs there is a small alveolar dead space in the erect posture, but this increases when alveoli are not perfused or when alveoli are overventilated in relation to their perfusion (fig 2.16). Pulmonary embolism obviously results in an increase in alveolar dead space, though the effects may be reduced by a concomitant reduction in ventilation to the affected area, induced by the local reduction in alveolar CO_2. A reduction in pulmonary artery pressure due to a decrease in cardiac output or to pulmonary vasodilator drugs will decrease perfusion in the non-dependent zones of the lung and may also result in a large increase in alveolar dead space. This may be accentuated if high alveolar pressures are generated by the ventilator when total ventilation is increased to compensate for the increase in alveolar dead space. Alveolar dead space may also increase when alveolar pressure is increased by the application of PEEP.

Alveoli with a high ratio of ventilation to perfusion also contribute to an increase in alveolar dead space because their CO_2 level is less than that in normal alveoli and so their ventilation removes less CO_2 per unit volume than normal. When patients with chronic lung disease develop ventilation-perfusion inequalities, the ratio of dead space to tidal volume increases and

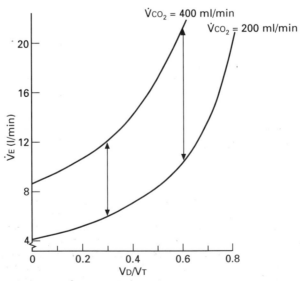

Fig 2.17 Minute volume ($\dot{V}E$) required to maintain normal arterial PCO_2 with different ratios of dead space to tidal volume (VD/VT) and a CO_2 production ($\dot{V}CO_2$) of 200 ml/min or 400 ml/min.

more ventilation is required to clear the CO_2 being produced. This is illustrated in fig 2.17. Few patients can sustain a minute ventilation of more than 12 l/min for prolonged periods so it is uncommon to see a patient breathing spontaneously with a dead space to tidal volume ratio of more than 0.6. Weaning from a mechanical ventilator is seldom successful when the ratio exceeds this value.

Effects of mechanical ventilation on gas distribution

Gravitationally induced changes in the shapes of the lungs and chest wall create a vertical gradient of pleural pressure, the pressure in the non-dependent part of the pleural space in the erect lung being about -1.0 kPa (-10 cm H_2O) whereas the pressure at the base is about -0.25 kPa

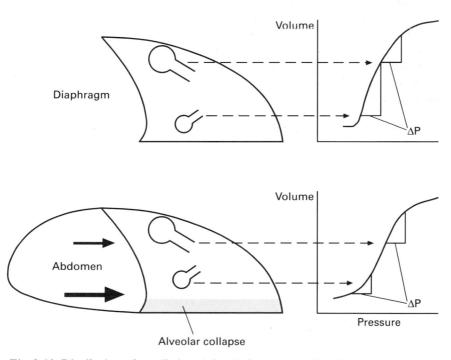

Fig 2.18 Distribution of ventilation. (above) Spontaneous breathing. Gravitationally induced gradient of pleural pressure causes non-dependent alveoli to be exposed to larger transpulmonary (distending) pressure than dependent alveoli at end of expiration. Because dependent alveoli are situated on a steeper portion of the pressure-volume curve, they will receive a greater proportion of tidal volume when transpulmonary pressure difference increases by a given increment of pressure (ΔP) during spontaneous inspiration. (below) Controlled ventilation. When diaphragm is inactive, hydrostatic pressure generated by abdominal contents decreases regional compliance of dependent zones, so diverting more ventilation to non-dependent zones. This effect may be accentuated by compression collapse of alveoli in dependent zones.

39

(-2.5 cm H_2O) with respect to atmospheric pressure. A similar, but smaller, gradient exists in the supine position. These differences in pleural pressure cause the alveoli in the non-dependent zones of the lungs to be exposed to a greater transpulmonary pressure difference than those in dependent lung zones (fig 2.18). As a result, the non-dependent alveoli have a larger resting volume than those in dependent zones. The dependent alveoli lie on a steeper part of the pressure-volume curve than non-dependent alveoli, but both are exposed to approximately the same increase in transpulmonary pressure during inspiration, so ventilation is delivered predominantly to the dependent lung zones in spontaneously breathing patients with normal lungs. This helps to match ventilation to the gravitational distribution of pulmonary blood flow (fig 2.19). During controlled ventilation with normal tidal volumes and frequencies, however, diaphragmatic activity is absent, and so the distribution of ventilation is influenced by the regional compliance of both the lung and the chest wall. When the patient is supine the liquid contents of the abdomen create a lateral pressure which forces the diaphragm up into the chest, the hydrostatic pressure being maximal in the dependent zones. This reduces FRC and causes ventilation to be distributed preferentially to the non-dependent zones of the lung; blood flow is still gravitationally determined, creating a major ventilation-perfusion mismatch, which results in an increase in alveolar dead space and venous admixture effect.

The induction of general anaesthesia or deep sedation results in a decrease

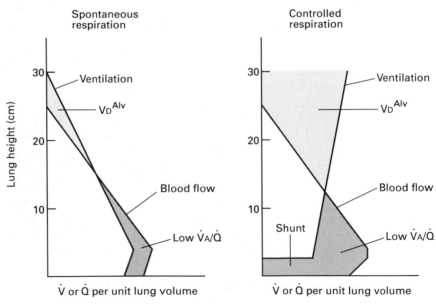

Fig 2.19 Blood flow ($\dot{Q}$) and ventilation ($\dot{V}$) plotted against lung height in the erect lung. (left) Normal distribution; (right) effects of anaesthesia and paralysis.

in functional residual capacity of 300–500 ml so that the resting positions of the upper and lower alveoli move downwards on the pressure-volume curve (fig 2.18). Anaesthesia also decreases the movement of the dependent parts of the diaphragm. This tends to decrease the ventilation in dependent zones during spontaneous ventilation and, in some circumstances, may induce dependent airway closure. If this occurs, ventilation to non-dependent zones may exceed that in dependent zones. In addition, anaesthesia causes compression collapse to develop in the most dependent zones of the lung. This occurs within a few minutes of induction in approximately 95% of patients; it is not abolished by the application of moderate positive end expiratory pressure and persists into the postoperative period.[19] Both of these factors tend to cause ventilation to be distributed preferentially to the non-dependent zones of the lung during spontaneous ventilation in anaesthetised patients, and the change in distribution is accentuated by the loss of diaphragmatic tone induced by muscle relaxant drugs and the use of controlled ventilation (fig 2.19).

In patients with normal lungs ventilated at normal tidal volumes and frequencies, the distribution of ventilation is governed mainly by regional compliance. However, variations in airway resistance may modify the distribution when high inspiratory flow rates are used, as this accentuates the pressure drops along the airways. The non-dependent alveoli and airways are more dilated than those in dependent zones and so they offer less resistance to flow – this may exaggerate the maldistribution produced by controlled ventilation when flow rates exceed 50–60 l/min. The effects are, however, much less than those produced by regional variations in airway resistance due to disease.

In patients with asthma or chronic obstructive airways disease, there are wide variations in regional time constants owing to changes in both compliance and resistance. Alveolar units with a short time constant (low resistance, low compliance, or both) will fill quickly but those with a long time constant (high resistance or high compliance) will fill slowly. If the ventilator is set to deliver a fixed tidal volume with a limited duration of inspiration, the alveoli with a long time constant will fail to achieve pressure equilibrium with mouth pressure, and so will be underventilated, whereas the alveoli with a short time constant will tend to be relatively overventilated. This results in an increase in both venous admixture and alveolar dead space. Although the maldistribution could theoretically be reduced by decreasing the breathing frequency, this is seldom possible because of the high minute volumes required to compensate for the increased alveolar dead space.

Effects of mechanical ventilation on the circulation

In 1948 Cournand and colleagues reported that cardiac output was decreased during mechanical ventilation and that the decrease was closely related to the increase in mean airway pressure.[20] It soon became apparent that the major cause of the decrease in cardiac output was a decrease in venous return associated with the increase in mean intrathoracic pressure resulting from the increase in airway pressure.[21] This mechanism may be augmented by an increase in pulmonary vascular resistance and effects on the heart when high airway pressures are used.

There is continuing debate concerning the relative importance of the various mechanisms involved. For example, an increase in pressure in the airways increases the transpulmonary pressure, which compresses the pulmonary capillaries but increases the diameter and length of the extra-alveolar vessels, so creating variable changes in pulmonary vascular resistance. Again, the expansion of the lung increases the absolute pressure in the pleural space, which decreases the gradient for venous return, but it also increases the pressure around the great vessels and heart, and this may affect preload and afterload. The situation is further complicated by changes in baroreceptor activity, by the influence of changes in arterial PO_2 and PCO_2 on myocardial contractility, and by the possible occurrence of myocardial ischaemia under certain conditions. The increase in arterial PO_2 resulting from the application of PEEP is also directly related to an increase in mean airway pressure,[22] so it can be seen that its beneficial effects on oxygenation may be counteracted by the decrease in cardiac output. Since these two opposing effects have to be carefully balanced when treating any patient with severe lung disease, it is important to understand how an increase in airway pressure may affect the circulation. To facilitate understanding, the changes will be considered under three headings; first, the cyclical changes associated with spontaneous ventilation; second, the factors which influence mean intrathoracic pressure; and third, the causes of the decrease in cardiac output during controlled ventilation.

Spontaneous versus controlled ventilation

During spontaneous breathing, the contraction of the inspiratory muscles produces a decrease in the absolute intrapleural pressure, which results in the expansion of the lungs; normally expiration results from the passive recoil of the lungs and chest wall. The 0.5–1 kPa (5–10 cm H_2O) decrease in absolute intrathoracic pressure during inspiration increases the gradient for venous return and so increases the transmural right atrial pressure, right ventricular preload, and stroke output. The decrease in pleural pressure also increases the transpulmonary pressure gradient, which tends to compress the pulmonary capillaries and so increase pulmonary vascular resistance and right ventricular afterload. However, the increase in afterload is relatively small when the lungs are normal and the patient breathes at normal tidal volumes, so the increased right ventricular output is transmitted to the left heart, where it increases left ventricular preload and stroke output. Since the onset

LEEDS METROPOLITAN UNIVERSITY LIBRARY

of the increased preload in the left ventricle occurs about three heartbeats after that in the right ventricle, left ventricular ejection and aortic pressure peak at the end of inspiration and beginning of expiration. The net effect is a transfer of blood from the periphery to the lungs during the early part of inspiration and the reverse during expiration.

When the same tidal volume is generated by IPPV similar changes in transpulmonary pressure occur, but the subatmospheric intrathoracic pressure increases towards atmospheric and even becomes positive with respect to atmospheric, so that venous return and right ventricular output are reduced during inspiration. Right ventricular ejection is further decreased by the small increase in afterload resulting from the lung inflation. However, the lung inflation squeezes some blood into the left atrium, and left ventricular afterload is decreased by the increase in pressure surrounding the left atrium and ventricle (since this augments the pressure difference between the ventricle and the major extrathoracic arteries). As a result, left ventricular ejection and aortic pressure tend to peak at the height of inspiration and then reach a minimum at the end of expiration.[23]

The oscillations in systolic arterial pressure which reflect the variations in left ventricular output between inspiration and expiration average about 10 mm Hg in the normovolaemic patient ventilated at normal tidal volumes. The magnitude of the oscillations is increased in the early stages of hypovolaemia.[24] It is also increased when tidal volume is increased or chest wall compliance is decreased, since these changes increase the magnitude of the swings in intrathoracic pressure. The oscillations are accentuated in the presence of a nodal rhythm but are usually minimal in patients who are hypervolaemic or in congestive cardiac failure.

Factors affecting mean intrathoracic pressure

IPPV and INPV. The circulatory effects produced by a given level of intermittent positive pressure or intermittent negative pressure ventilation are identical, for both techniques decrease the pressure gradient for venous return during inspiration, so that cardiac output is decreased. The difference between the two is that with IPPV the intrathoracic pressure is increased while the pressure around the peripheral veins remains constant, but with a tank ventilator the pressure at the mouth remains constant while the pressure surrounding the veins decreases, due to the generation of a subatmospheric pressure within the tank. The only circumstance when INPV does not interfere with the circulation is when the pressure change is limited to the thorax by the use of a cuirass.[25] The intrathoracic pressure is then decreased by the outward pull of the chest wall during inspiration, but the pressure around the peripheral veins is unchanged. Unfortunately, it is difficult to obtain an airtight fit between the cuirass and the chest wall, so most cuirass

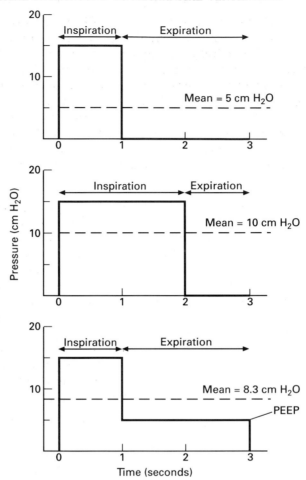

Fig 2.20 Effects of changes of inspiration: expiration (I:E) ratio and of adding positive end expiratory pressure (PEEP) on mean airway pressure. (top) I:E = 1:2; (centre) I:E = 2:1; (bottom) I:E = 1:2 with PEEP.

ventilators are relatively inefficient; they are therefore generally used to provide ventilatory assistance for patients with limited ventilatory capacity.

Mean airway pressure. In normal individuals the mean intrathoracic pressure is closely related to the mean airway pressure. It is impossible to estimate mean airway pressure from the standard aneroid gauge on the ventilator and difficult to do so even if a dynamic trace is available, but many ventilators now provide a digital readout of both dynamic and mean airway pressures. Mean airway pressure depends on peak inspiratory pressure, the duration of inspiration and expiration, and the shape of the inspiratory and expiratory pressure wave forms. Fig 2.20 shows how an increase in the duration of inspiration or the presence of PEEP during expiration can increase mean airway pressure, even though the peak airway pressure remains the same. Theoretically, for any given inspiratory period and tidal volume, a descending flow waveform (which fills the lung early in inspiration) should produce a higher mean intrathoracic pressure than an ascending flow waveform, and sine and square waveforms should yield intermediate values (fig 2.14). However, the patterns originated by the ventilator are downgraded during their transmission to the pleural space and it is usually not possible to detect any difference in mean intrathoracic pressure when waveforms are changed, providing that the tidal volume and inspiratory period are identical.[26]

Mean alveolar pressure. Although mean airway pressure may be measured at the mouth, this may provide a poor indication of the pressure existing in the alveoli, as equilibrium between mouth and alveolar pressures occurs only under zero flow conditions. During inspiration the airway pressure exceeds the alveolar pressure because some of the airway pressure is used to overcome the airway resistance; during expiration there is a gradient of pressure in the opposite direction. When airway resistance is low, mean airway pressure provides a reasonable approximation to mean alveolar pressure. However, when airway resistance is increased there may be an appreciable difference between the two. Under such circumstances expiration may be prolonged by the increased resistance, and sometimes by dynamic narrowing of the airways, so that the alveoli remain inflated by the intrinsic PEEP and mean alveolar pressure may exceed mean airway pressure (fig 2.9).

Lung compliance. During a positive pressure inspiration only a proportion of the increased alveolar pressure is transmitted to the pleural space.[27] As the compliances of the lung and chest wall are normally equal, the change in pleural pressure during lung inflation is approximately half the change in alveolar pressure. In patients with emphysema, however, where lung compliance is increased, up to 70% of the change in alveolar pressure may be transmitted to the pleural space. Similarly, a reduction in lung compliance may reduce transmission so that the change in pleural pressure is only 30% of that in the alveoli. This explains why high peak airway pressures may have surprisingly little effect on the circulation in some patients. This factor is particularly important in the treatment of the neonatal respiratory distress syndrome – high airway pressures are often required in the early stages, when surfactant is deficient, and failure to reduce the airway pressure during recovery may result in severe circulatory problems.

Regional variations in compliance may cause pressures around the heart, for example, to differ from those in the rest of the pleural space. Changes in intrathoracic pressure are rarely measured directly in clinical practice, but a useful indication of their magnitude is provided by the respiratory oscillations on the central venous pressure trace.

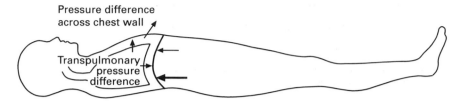

Fig 2.21 Determinants of pleural pressure. Transpulmonary pressure difference depends on tidal volume and lung compliance. Pressure difference across chest wall depends on tidal volume and on chest wall compliance, which may be influenced by abdominal distension, particularly if the diaphragm is paralysed.

Chest wall compliance. As shown in fig 2.21, the two factors that determine the tidal variation in pleural pressure are tidal volume and chest wall compliance. The latter may be reduced by obesity, kyphoscoliosis, thoracic burns, distension of the abdominal contents, encircling bandages, or strapping. (A surgeon leaning on the chest during a lengthy operation produces similar effects.) An increase in end expiratory lung volume due to increased airway resistance will also result in an appreciable increase in mean intrathoracic pressure. This is particularly important during mechanical ventilation, since caval flow normally increases during expiration to compensate for the decrease in flow during lung inflation. In patients with severe airways obstruction there may be an increase in expiratory muscle activity and this may further increase intrathoracic pressure during expiration. These factors account for much of the difficulty in maintaining an adequate cardiac output in patients who are mechanically ventilated for the treatment of a severe attack of asthma.

Causes of decreased cardiac output

An increase in airway pressure may reduce cardiac output in three ways. The most important is a reduction in venous return. Effects of increased airways pressure on the pulmonary circulation and heart become important only at higher levels of pressure.[28]

Venous return. The major cause of the reduction of cardiac output during controlled mechanical ventilation is the decrease in venous return resulting from the increase in intrathoracic pressure. The magnitude of the decrease in cardiac output depends, firstly, on the mean intrathoracic pressure, which affects the transmural or filling pressure of the heart, and, secondly, on the peripheral venous pressure. The mean intrathoracic pressure is usually closely related to the increase in mean airway pressure and so depends on the peak pressure, the inspiratory:expiratory (I:E) time ratio, the shape of the applied inspiratory waveform, and the presence of any positive alveolar

Circulatory effects of increased alveolar pressure

At all airway pressures:

Reduction in venous return due to increased mean intrathoracic pressure
  Can be restored by increasing peripheral venous pressure

At high airway pressures:

Increased pulmonary vascular resistance
  Induces compensatory increase in right ventricular end diastolic volume (but
  this may cause decrease in left ventricular end diastolic volume due to
  deviation of interventricular septum, and may cause compression of coronary
  vessels in wall of right ventricle)

Increased pressure around heart
  May help to unload myocardium in patients with heart failure

pressure during expiration. The peripheral venous pressure depends on posture, blood volume, and peripheral venous tone. The decrease in cardiac output resulting from the application of PEEP can be minimised by raising the legs, applying an antigravity suit, administering venoconstrictor drugs, or increasing blood volume,[29] but it is important to control these manoeuvres by measurements of central venous or pulmonary wedge pressure to ensure that the heart is not overloaded, for heart failure may be precipitated if PEEP is suddenly removed.[30] Normally, a cyclical increase in sympathetic tone partially compensates for the increase in intrathoracic pressure during the inspiratory phase of IPPV, but this is less effective if the venous system is already constricted to compensate for a decreased blood volume.[31] Furthermore, this mechanism may be less efficient or absent in patients with an autonomic neuropathy due to diseases such as diabetes or the Guillain-Barré syndrome. Such patients often suffer profound reductions in cardiac output when connected to the ventilator, and they may need volume expansion or vasoconstrictor drugs to maintain an adequate arterial pressure.

The pulmonary circulation. Changes in pulmonary vascular resistance with lung volume are complicated by the fact that the pulmonary circulation is composed of both intra-alveolar and extra-alveolar vessels, which differ in their response to lung inflation. The intra-alveolar vessels are the pulmonary capillaries which normally contribute about 40% of the total pulmonary vascular resistance. They are directly in contact with the pressure in the alveoli and are compressed when transpulmonary pressure is increased, whether the inspiration is spontaneous or controlled (fig 2.22). Because of the gravitational distribution of pulmonary blood flow, an increase in transpulmonary pressure will initially result in the cessation of blood flow in the non-

47

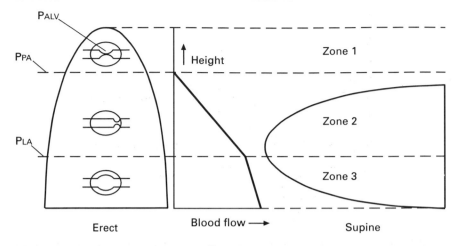

Fig 2.22 Three zone model of the lung.[32] In erect posture, pulmonary capillaries in zone 1 are collapsed since alveolar pressure (PALV) exceeds pulmonary artery pressure (PPA) and left atrial pressure (PLA). The size of this zone will increase if alveolar pressure is increased or pulmonary artery pressure is reduced. In supine posture, vertical height of lung is less and there is no zone 1.

dependent parts of the lungs, but as the pressure is increased the level of capillary closure will move down the lung, thereby increasing the volume of West's zone 1, and increasing the alveolar dead space.[32] The resulting reduction in perfused vascular bed will increase right ventricular afterload. This will increase right ventricular end diastolic volume and right ventricular stroke volume and result in an increase in pulmonary artery pressure, so tending to restore the volume of perfused lung.

The extra-alveolar vessels consist of the major vessels entering or leaving the lung and the remainder of the vessels within the lung parenchyma. The major vessels are exposed directly to the pleural pressure and are probably expanded by a spontaneous inspiration but compressed when absolute pleural pressure is increased during a positive pressure inspiration. However, the vessels within the lung are held open by the elastic recoil of the adjacent lung tissue and so increase in diameter when the lung is expanded, whether the inspiration is spontaneous or controlled. They narrow when lung volume is reduced. The combined effects of these two sets of vessels results in a U shaped curve of pulmonary vascular resistance against lung volume, with resistance being minimal at the FRC, but increasing steeply at lower and higher lung volumes (fig 2.23). The net effect of a positive pressure inflation on pulmonary vascular resistance will therefore depend on the initial volume of the lung and on the changes in transpulmonary pressure and tidal volume.

It used to be thought that an increase in resistance of the extra-alveolar vessels accounted for part of the reduction in blood flow in collapsed areas of

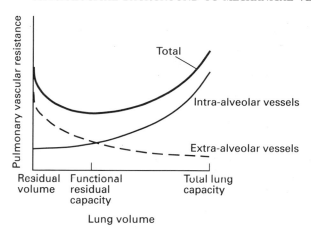

Fig 2.23 Variation of resistance of intra-alveolar and extra-alveolar vessels resistance with lung volume.

lung, but it now seems clear that the reduction in flow is due almost entirely to hypoxic pulmonary vasoconstriction augmented by equilibration with the higher PCO_2 of the mixed venous blood.[33]

The evidence suggests that in patients with relatively normal lungs given IPPV, peak inflation pressures up to 10–15 cm H_2O produce little change in pulmonary vascular resistance, changes in cardiac output being due largely to the effects of the increased intrathoracic pressure on venous return. However, when lung disease is present high airway pressures may be required, and these may have major effects on right ventricular afterload, particularly if pulmonary vascular resistance is already increased.[34] Hyperinflation in patients with chronic obstructive lung disease and asthma may also increase right ventricular afterload. The pulmonary hypertension seen in many patients with severe acute lung disease increases right ventricular work and oxygen consumption and may lead to myocardial ischaemia if myocardial blood flow is limited. Whereas left coronary flow depends predominantly on aortic diastolic pressure, right coronary flow occurs in both systole and diastole. It is therefore essential to maintain an adequate systolic arterial pressure in such patients in order to ensure that right ventricular subendocardial blood flow is maintained at optimal levels.

The heart. High airway pressures may have other complex effects on the heart and circulation. The increase in right ventricular pressure resulting from the increased pulmonary vascular resistance may cause the interventricular septum to bulge into the left ventricle, so decreasing left ventricular compliance and left ventricular stroke output.[35] On the other hand, in patients with heart failure, the increase in pressure around the heart may

49

unload the left ventricle and so improve the efficiency of contraction.[36] This contrasts with the situation when there are large negative intrathoracic pressure swings during spontaneous respiration in patients with upper airway obstruction or asthma, for these may increase left ventricular afterload.[37] Studies on the effects of positive pressure ventilation on the heart have yielded variable results, probably because of regional differences in the transmission of pressure due to regional differences in compliance and the presence or absence of heart disease.

There are many other explanations for the reduction in cardiac output during high levels of PEEP.[38] Most suggest that there is a reduction in left ventricular end diastolic volume, but whether this is due to external pressure from the distended lungs or due to altered pressure-volume characteristics of the left ventricle is not clear.

Other effects on the circulation. The haemodynamic effects of mechanical ventilation may be modified by the changes in arterial blood gases resulting from its use. For example, a decrease in arterial PCO_2 due to hyperventilation will decrease the sympathetic drive to the heart and so reduce cardiac output.[39] An increase in PCO_2 may cause dysrhythmias which, if severe enough, may have a similar effect. PCO_2 levels also affect regional circulations. For example, the cerebral circulation is extremely sensitive to changes in PCO_2, and an increase may lead to a considerable increase in cerebral blood flow and intracranial pressure. Similarly, a sudden decrease in PCO_2 in a patient who has had a longstanding hypercapnia due to chronic obstructive airways disease may cause cerebral ischaemia and convulsions.

The change in arterial PO_2 resulting from the application of PEEP may also affect the regional circulations and oxygen transport to the tissues. Oxygen transport will be increased only if the increase in arterial oxgyen content produced by the PEEP is great enough to offset the almost invariable decrease in cardiac output resulting from its use. This is seldom achieved unless the initial oxygen saturation is below 85–90%.

Finally, it must be remembered that the increase in mean intrathoracic and peripheral venous pressure associated with mechanical ventilation, and particularly with PEEP, may affect the distribution of fluid between the intravascular and extravascular compartments and so lead to peripheral oedema and decreases in blood volume. The increased venous pressure may also increase intracranial pressure and cause a deterioration in the condition of patients with a head injury.

Effects of PEEP on the circulation. The application of PEEP increases peak and mean intrathoracic pressure during both inspiration and expiration, a given level of PEEP producing a corresponding increase in mean airway pressure. Thus, even low levels of PEEP result in appreciable increases in mean alveolar and intrathoracic pressure, which decrease venous return and so decrease cardiac output. An increase in blood volume will usually restore cardiac output towards normal levels when PEEP levels are less than 10–15 cm H_2O, but such an increase may have only a limited effect at higher levels because of complex effects on the lungs and the heart.

PEEP is usually used to recruit collapsed alveoli when there is severe arterial hypoxaemia despite the administration of high concentrations of oxygen. However, the effect of PEEP on pulmonary vascular resistance depends on the state of the lungs when it is applied. It has already been pointed out that in the normal lung pulmonary vascular resistance is at a minimum at the FRC, and that both increased and decreased lung volume result in a increased resistance. Alveolar collapse results in a decrease in FRC and in hypoxic vasoconstriction, the latter resulting in a reduction in blood flow to hypoxic areas of up to 50%. When PEEP is applied, it is distributed preferentially to ventilated areas of lung, where it compresses the pulmonary capillaries and so causes an increase in resistance. This tends to drive blood into the non-ventilated areas of lung, so tending to increase the intrapulmonary shunt. However, if PEEP recruits previously collapsed areas of lung without producing a significant increase in resistance in ventilated areas, it should produce a reduction in shunt and a decrease in pulmonary vascular resistance due to the abolition of hypoxic vasoconstriction.

It will be apparent that the effects of PEEP on pulmonary vascular resistance are complex, but they will inevitably increase right ventricular afterload. Right ventricular work will be increased, and this may lead to myocardial ischaemia, particularly if arterial pressure is low or there is severe arterial hypoxaemia.

Harmful effects of PEEP

Increases peak airway pressure: leads to pulmonary barotrauma

Increases mean airway pressure:
  May increase alveolar dead space
  May increase shunt by diverting blood flow to non-ventilated areas of lung

Increases mean intrathoracic pressure: decreases cardiac output

Increases central venous pressure:
  Shifts fluid from intravascular to extravascular compartments
  Produces congestion in gastrointestinal tract and possibly increases risk of bleeding
  Decreases blood flow and may impair function in other organs (decreased urine flow)
  May also decrease thoracic duct lymph flow and hinder absorption of pulmonary oedema

Increases cerebrospinal fluid pressure:
  May impair cerebral circulation

Effects of PEEP on the kidney and other organs

Kidney

The possible effect of an increase in intrathoracic pressure on renal function was first noted in 1947.[40] Since then there have been many reports documenting a reduction in urine output and sodium excretion in response to the application of PEEP.[41] These effects are smaller with CPAP than with mechanical ventilation and PEEP.[42] They are probably due mainly to haemodynamic changes but may also be due to sympathetic stimulation and hormonal responses.

The increase in mean intrathoracic pressure affects the kidney in two ways: it decreases cardiac output and arterial pressure, and it increases the pressure in the renal vein. It seems unlikely that a reduction in arterial pressure is responsible for the changes in renal function because the kidney has an autoregulatory mechanism that functions efficiently down to a systolic pressure of about 75 mm Hg. However, a reduction in cardiac output decreases renal perfusion, particularly renal cortical flow, and this results in a decrease in glomerular filtration rate.[43] A reduction in cortical flow and increased medullary flow would also explain the reduction in sodium excretion since the juxtamedullary nephrons tend to retain sodium to a greater extent than cortical nephrons.[44] The decrease in cardiac output is not the sole cause of the renal changes because it has been shown that restoring cardiac output by increasing blood volume during the application of 12 cm H_2O PEEP fails to restore urine output to normal levels.[30] It is possible that renal haemodynamics are also affected by the increase in renal vein pressure, for it has been shown that vena caval constriction can decrease glomerular filtration rate and decrease sodium excretion.[45] A change in the distribution of renal blood flow has also been found in patients in heart failure.[46]

A decrease in transaortic pressure may also decrease baroreceptor stimulation and so increase renal sympathetic activity. For example, dogs with an intact nervous system show the expected decrease in renal function with increased intrathoracic pressure but dogs with denervated carotid baroreceptors show no change in renal function.[47]

Another possibility is that the changes in renal function may be partially mediated by the secretion of antidiuretic hormone.[48] The evidence is conflicting, partly because secretion of the hormone is affected by changes in the blood gases, and partly because the response seems to vary with the respiratory pattern used. Thus, although urinary flow and glomerular filtration rate are both decreased by controlled mechanical ventilation with PEEP and spontaneous breathing with CPAP, only the former causes an increase in plasma concentrations of the hormone and a decrease in urinary sodium concentration.[41] In a recent study in patients, Payen and colleagues failed to find any increase in secretion of the hormone.[49] The renin-angiotensin system and atrial natriuretic factor may also be involved in the changes.[48, 50]

Liver

The reduction of cardiac output associated with the use of PEEP produces a corresponding reduction on global hepatic flow, which can be reversed by blood volume expansion.[51] Hepatic flow may also be reduced by increasing hepatic vascular resistance. This could be due to an increase in caval pressure or to mechanical compression of the liver by the diaphragm or by the increase in intra-abdominal pressure.[52, 53]

Gastrointestinal system

Gastrointestinal bleeding is a not uncommon complication of mechanical ventilation in severely ill patients in the intensive care unit. This bleeding could be caused by the combination of the increase in venous pressure and decrease in cardiac output associated with PEEP. The incidence of bleeding is reduced by the prophylactic administration of H_2 blocking drugs, so it seems likely that other factors may be important.

Conclusions

Although controlled ventilation can produce significant improvements in gas exchange and acid-base balance, it induces a series of physiological changes that may, in the short or long term, prove deleterious for the patient. There is some evidence that techniques which permit the patient to breathe spontaneously for part or all of the time reduce the magnitude of some of these disturbances. However, the pattern of ventilation in patients with respiratory failure differs from normal spontaneous respiration, and it may well be that spontaneous respiration may prove beneficial only when the respiratory pattern is not distorted by fatigue or an excessive respiratory drive.

1 Pride NB. The assessment of airflow obstruction. Role of measurements of airways resistance and tests of forced expiration. *Br J Dis Chest* 1971;65:136–69.
2 Bolder PM, Healy TEJ, Bolder AR, Beatty PCW, Kay B. The extra work of breathing through adult endotracheal tubes. *Anesth Analg* 1986;65:853–9.
3 Wright PE, Marini JJ, Bernard GR. *In vitro* versus *in vivo* comparison of endotracheal tube airflow resistance. *Am Rev Respir Dis* 1989;140:10–16.
4 Gottfried SB, Reissman H, Ranieri VM. A simple method for the measurement of intrinsic positive end-expiratory pressure during controlled and assisted modes of mechanical ventilation. *Crit Care Med* 1992;20:621–9.
5 Smith TC, Marini JJ. Impact of PEEP on lung mechanics and work of breathing in severe airflow obstruction. *J Appl Physiol* 1988;65:1488–99.
6 Pesenti A, Pelosi P, Rossi N, Virtuani A, Brazzi L, Rossi A. The effects of positive end-

expiratory pressure on respiratory resistance in patients with the adult respiratory distress syndrome and in normal anesthetized subjects. *Am Rev Respir Dis* 1991;**144**:101–7.

7 Eberhard L, Guttmann J, Wolff W, Bertschmann W, Minzer A, Kohl H-J, *et al*. Intrinsic PEEP monitored in the ventilated ARDS patient with a mathematical method. *J Appl Physiol* 1992;**73**:479–85.

8 Sykes MK. Respiratory mechanics. In: Scurr C, Feldman S, Soni N, eds. *Scientific foundations of anaesthesia. The basis of intensive care.* 4th ed. Oxford: Heinemann Medical, 1990:254–72.

9 Matamis D, Lemaire F, Harf A, Brun-Buisson C, Ansquer JC, Atlan G. Total respiratory pressure-volume curves in the adult respiratory distress syndrome. *Chest* 1984;**86**:58–66.

10 Mankikian B, Lemaire F, Benito S, Brun-Buisson C, Harf A, Maillot JP, *et al*. A new device for measurement of pulmonary pressure-volume curves in patients on mechanical ventilation. *Crit Care Med* 1983;**11**:897–901.

11 Gattinoni L, Mascheroni D, Basilico E, Foti G, Pesenti A, Avalli L. Volume/pressure curve of total respiratory system in paralyzed patients: artefacts and correction factors. *Intensive Care Med* 1987;**13**:19–25.

12 Gattinoni L, Pesenti A, Avalli L, Rossi F, Bombino M. Pressure-volume curve of total respiratory system in acute respiratory failure. Computed tomographic scan study. *Am Rev Respir Dis* 1987;**136**:730–6.

13 Mathe JC, Clement A, Chevalier JY, Gaultier C, Costil J. Use of total inspiratory pressure-volume curves for determination of appropriate positive end-expiratory pressure in newborns with hyaline membrane disease. *Intensive Care Med* 1987;**13**:332–6.

14 Fernández R, Mancebo J, Blanch LI, Benito S, Calaf N, Net A. Intrinsic PEEP on static pressure-volume curves. *Intensive Care Med* 1990;**16**:233–6.

15 Korst RJ, Orlando R, Yeston NS, Molin M, de Graff AC, Gluck E. Validation of respiratory mechanics software in microprocessor-controlled ventilators. *Crit Care Med* 1992;**20**:1152–6.

16 Sydow M, Burchardi H, Zinserling J, Ische H, Crozier Th A, Weyland W. Improved determination of static compliance by automated single volume steps in ventilated patients. *Intensive Care Med* 1991;**17**:108–14.

17 Sydow M, Burchardi H, Zinserling J, Crozier Th A, Denecke T, Zielmann S. Intrinsic PEEP determined by static pressure-volume curves – application of a novel automated occlusion method. *Intensive Care Med* 1993;**19**:166–71.

18 Covelli HD, Black JW, Olsen MS, Beekman JF. Respiratory failure precipitated by high carbohydrate loads. *Ann Intern Med* 1981;**95**:579–81.

19 Lindberg P, Gunnarsson L, Tokics L, Secher E, Lundquist H, Brismar B, *et al*. Atelectasis and lung function in the postoperative period. *Acta Anaesthesiol Scand* 1992;**36**:546–53.

20 Cournand A, Motley HL, Werko L, Richards DW. Physiological studies of the effect of intermittent positive pressure breathing on cardiac output in man. *Am J Physiol* 1948;**152**:162–74.

21 Morgan BC, Martin WE, Hornbein TF, Crawford EW, Guntheroth WG. Hemodynamic effects of intermittent positive pressure respiration. *Anesthesiology* 1966;**27**:584–90.

22 Pesenti A, Marcolin R, Prato P, Borelli M, Riboni A, Gattinoni L. Mean airway pressure vs positive end-expiratory pressure during mechanical ventilation. *Crit Care Med* 1985;**13**:34–7.

23 Jardin F, Farcot J-C, Gueret P, Prost J-F, Ozier Y, Bourdarias J-P. Cyclic changes in arterial pulse during respiratory support. *Circulation* 1983;**68**:266–74.

24 Szold A, Pizof R, Segal E, Perel A. The effect of tidal volume and intravascular volume state on systolic pressure variation in ventilated dogs. *Intensive Care Med* 1989;**15**:368–71.

25 Ambrosino N, Cobelli F, Torbicki A, Opasich C, Pozzoli M, Fracchia C, *et al*. Hemodynamic effects of negative-pressure ventilation in patients with COPD. *Chest* 1990;**97**:850–6.

26 Johansson H. Effect of different gas flow patterns on central circulation during respirator treatment. *Acta Anaesthesiol Scand* 1975;**19**:96–103.

27 Jardin F, Genevray B, Brun-Ney D, Bourdarias J-P. Influence of lung and chest wall compliance on transmission of airway pressure to the pleural space in critically ill patients. *Chest* 1985;**88**:653–8.

28 Sharf SM, Brown R, Saunders N, Green LH. Hemodynamic effects of positive-pressure inflation. *J Appl Physiol* 1980;**49**:124–31.

29 Sykes MK, Adams AP, Finlay WEI, McCormick PW, Economides A. The effects of end-

expiratory inflation pressure on cardiorespiratory function in normo-, hypo-, and hypervolaemic dogs. *Br J Anaesth* 1970;**42**:669–77.

30 Qvist J, Pontoppidan H, Wilson RS, Lowenstein E, Laver MB. Hemodynamic responses to mechanical ventilation with PEEP: the effect of hypervolemia. *Anesthesiology* 1975;**42**:45–55.

31 Selldén H, Sjövall H, Wallin BG, Häggendal J, Ricksten S-E. Changes in muscle sympathetic nerve activity, venous plasma catecholamines, and calf vascular resistance during mechanical ventilation with PEEP in humans. *Anesthesiology* 1989;**70**:243–50.

32 West JB. *Regional differences in the lung.* London: Academic Press, 1977.

33 McFarlane PA, Gardaz J-P, Sykes MK. CO_2 and mechanical factors reduce blood flow in a collapsed lung lobe. *J Appl Physiol* 1984;**57**:739–43.

34 Jardin F, Delorme G, Hardy A, Auvert B, Beauchet A, Bourdarias J-P. Reevaluation of hemodynamic consequences of positive pressure ventilation: emphasis on cyclic right ventricular afterloading by mechanical lung inflation. *Anesthesiology* 1990;**72**:966–70.

35 Jardin JF, Farcot J-C, Boisante L, Curien N, Margairaz A, Bourdarias J-P. Influence of positive end-expiratory pressure on left ventricular performance. *N Engl J Med* 1981;**304**:387–92.

36 Mathru M, Rao TLK, El-Etr AA, Pifarre R. Hemodynamic response to changes in ventilatory patterns in patients with normal and poor left ventricular reserve. *Crit Care Med* 1982;**10**:423–6.

37 Buda AG, Pinsky MR, Ingels NB, Daughters GT, Stinson EB, Alderman EL. Effect of intrathoracic pressure on left ventricular performance. *N Engl J Med* 1979;**301**:453–9.

38 Tyler DC. Positive end-expiratory pressure: a review. *Crit Care Med* 1983;**11**:300–8.

39 Prys-Roberts C, Kelman GR, Greenbaum R, Robinson RH. Circulatory influences of artificial ventilation during nitrous oxide anaesthesia in man. II. Results: the relative influence of mean intrathoracic pressure and arterial carbon dioxide tension. *Br J Anaesth* 1967;**39**:533–48.

40 Drury DR, Henry JP, Goodman J. The effects of continuous positive pressure breathing on kidney function. *J Clin Invest* 1947;**26**:945–51.

41 Sladen A, Laver MB, Pontoppidan H. Pulmonary complications and water retention in prolonged mechanical ventilation. *N Engl J Med* 1968;**279**:448–53.

42 Marquez JM, Douglas ME, Downs JB, Wu W-H, Mantini EL, Kuck EJ, *et al.* Renal function and cardiovascular responses during positive airway pressure. *Anesthesiology* 1979;**50**:393–8.

43 Gammanpila S, Bevan DR, Bhudu R. Effect of positive and negative expiratory pressure on renal function. *Br J Anaesth* 1977;**49**:199–205.

44 Hall SV, Johnson EE, Hedley-Whyte J. Renal hemodynamics and function with continuous positive-pressure ventilation in dogs. *Anesthesiology* 1974;**41**:452–61.

45 Schrier RW, Humphreys MH. Factors involved in the natriuretic effects of acute constriction of the thoracic and abdominal inferior vena cava. *Circ Res* 1971;**29**:479–89.

46 Kilkoyne MM, Schmidt DH, Cannon PJ. Intrarenal blood flow in congestive heart failure. *Circulation* 1973;**47**:786–97.

47 Fewell JE, Bond GC. Role of sinoaortic baroreceptors in initiating the renal response to continuous positive pressure ventilation in the dog. *Anesthesiology* 1980;**52**:408–13.

48 Annat G, Viale JP, Bui Xuan B, Hadj Aissa O, Benzoni D, Vincent M, *et al.* Effect of PEEP ventilation on renal function, plasma renin, aldosterone, neurophysins and urinary ADH, and prostaglandins. *Anesthesiology* 1983;**58**:136–41.

49 Payen D, Farge D, Beloucif S, Leviel F, De La Cossaye JE, Carli P, *et al.* No involvement of ADH in acute antidiuresis during PEEP ventilation in humans. *Anesthesiology* 1987;**66**:17–23.

50 Kharasch ED, Yeo K-T, Kenny MA, Buffington CH. Atrial natriuretic factor may mediate the renal effects of PEEP ventilation. *Anesthesiology* 1988;**69**:862–9.

51 Matuschak GM, Pinsky MR, Rogers RM. Effects of positive end-expiratory pressure on hepatic blood flow and performance. *J Appl Physiol* 1987;**62**:1377–83.

52 Johnson EE, Hedley-Whyte J. Continuous positive-pressure ventilation and choledochoduodenal flow resistance. *J Appl Physiol* 1975;**39**:937–42.

53 Johnson EE, Hedley-Whyte J. Continuous positive-pressure ventilation and portal flow in dogs with pulmonary edema. *J Appl Physiol* 1972;**33**:385–9.

3 The mechanical basis of respiratory support

This chapter deals with the basic mechanical principles used in apparatus designed to provide respiratory support and traces the development of machines to the present day. The machines most commonly used in current practice are described in more detail in chapter 6. A fuller analysis of the construction and functional characteristics of past and present ventilators is given in other publications.[1-4]

Classification of ventilators

Several methods have been used to classify ventilators,[5] but the most satisfactory system is that devised by Mapleson.[6] This analysis ignores both the mechanical design of the ventilator and the source of its motive power, but classifies the machine according to its functional characteristics. The advantages of this method of classification are, firstly, that the behaviour of the machine under different clinical circumstances can be accurately predicted, and, secondly, that imperfections in the machine can be readily detected by tests on a model lung. Two aspects of function are considered: the way in which the ventilator controls the pattern of gas flow in and out of the patient (the driving mechanisms), and the mechanisms which cause the ventilator to cycle between the two phases of respiration (the cycling mechanisms) (table 3.1).

Table 3.1 Classification of ventilators
(I = inspiration; E = expiration)

Driving mechanisms	Cycling mechanisms	
Inspiratory phase	I to E	E to I

Flow generator:
   Constant
   Variable
	Time
	 Pressure
		Time
		 Patient

Pressure generator:
   Constant
   Variable
	Volume
	 Flow
	 Mixed
		Mixed

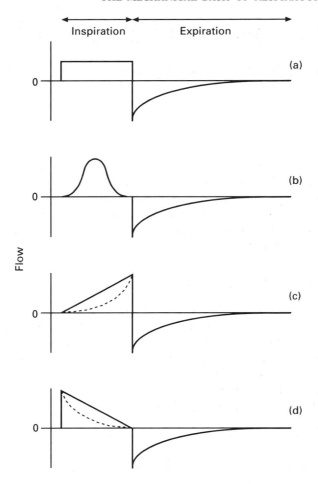

Fig 3.1 Common types of inspiratory flow pattern produced by flow generator: (a) constant (square wave); (b) sine wave; (c) ascending ramp; (d) descending ramp. The dotted lines in (c) and (d) are accelerating and decelerating flow patterns. Expiration is passive, the lungs behaving as a pressure generator, so that alveolar pressure and expiratory flow decrease approximately exponentially.

Driving mechanisms

Flow generators. The first characteristic, the method by which the gas is driven into the patient, divides ventilators into two groups – flow generators and pressure generators. The classification is based solely on the results of the interaction between the ventilator driving mechanism and the impedances to respiration produced by the lungs and chest wall. If the driving mechanism generates a fixed pattern of flow that is maintained despite changes in airway

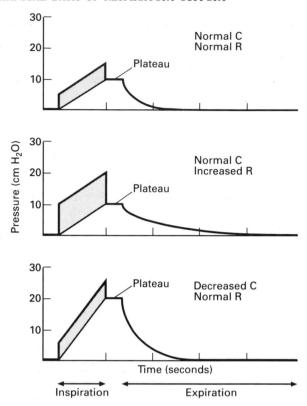

Fig 3.2 Effects of changes in airway resistance (R) and compliance (C) on airway pressure during ventilation with constant flow generator. Tidal volume = 1000 ml, inspiratory time = 1 s, pause time = 0.3 s. (top) $C = 1 \, l \, kPa^{-1}$ (0.1 l/cm H_2O); $R = 0.5 \, kPa \, l^{-1} \, s$ (5 cm H_2O/l/s). (centre) compliance unchanged, resistance doubled; (bottom) compliance halved, resistance unchanged.

resistance and compliance, the ventilator is classified as a flow generator. It does not matter whether the pattern of flow is constant throughout inspiration or whether it follows a sine wave, ascending ramp, descending ramp, or any other pattern (fig 3.1). What matters is whether that pattern is maintained in the face of a change of compliance or resistance. In a perfect flow generator changes in compliance and resistance have no effect on the flow pattern, but changes in airway pressure inevitably occur (fig 3.2). Although few ventilators are capable of maintaining the set flow pattern against large changes in compliance or resistance, it is important to monitor changes in airway pressure when using a flow generator, for these provide a useful guide to changes in the lung.

If the tidal volume and duration of inspiration are known it is a simple matter to calculate the inspiratory flow rate with a constant flow generator.

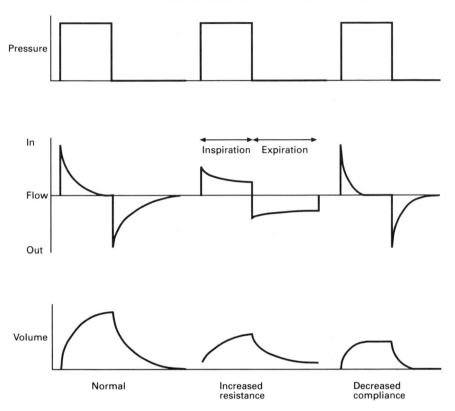

Fig 3.3 Recordings of airway pressure, flow, and lung volume with constant pressure generator: (left) normal resistance and compliance; (centre) increased resistance, normal compliance; (right) normal resistance, decreased compliance. Note that increased resistance results in decrease in tidal volume when inspiratory time is limited. It may also lead to incomplete emptying of lung and development of intrinsic PEEP.

For example, if a tidal volume of 500 ml is produced by an inspiration of 1 second, the flow rate must be 500 ml/second or 30 l/min. It is more difficult to calculate the peak flow rate for other patterns of flow. Fortunately, manufacturers tend to restrict the flow patterns to well known geometric shapes such as a sine wave or an ascending or descending ramp (fig 3.1). For the same tidal volume and duration of inspiration, peak flow with a ramp waveform is twice that of a constant flow generator; peak flow with a sine wave is 1.57 times the square wave flow rate. The ascending and descending ramp patterns are often wrongly referred to as accelerating or decelerating waveforms. The differences between the latter and the ramp waveforms are illustrated in figure 3.1.

59

Pressure generators. A pressure generator differs from a flow generator in that it generates a relatively low pressure (which again may be constant or may vary in a defined pattern), but the flow that results depends on the pattern of pressure and on the resistance and compliance encountered as the gas flows into the lungs. With a constant pressure generator the difference in pressure between the ventilator and alveoli will be maximal at the beginning of inspiration – flow will also be maximal at this time and will then decrease exponentially (fig 3.3). As discussed in chapter 2, the pattern of an exponential change can be characterised by the time constant (T), and in the normal lung this can be calculated from the product of its compliance (C) and resistance (R):

$$T = C \times R = 0.1 \ 1 \ kPa^{-1} \times 0.2 \ kPa \ l^{-1} \ s = 0.2 \ s$$

so the filling of the lung should be 95% complete in 0.6 s and 99% complete in 0.8 s. With an inspiratory time of 1 second and an expiratory time of 2 seconds flow should be close to zero at the end of each phase. However, if the time constant is increased to 1 second by an increase in airway resistance to 1 kPa l^{-1} s the filling of the lung will be only 63% complete at the end of a 1 second inspiration, and tidal volume will decrease. Expiration will also be incomplete, so that end expiratory lung volume will increase (fig 3.3). Within a few breaths a new equilibrium will have been established in which the

---

Ventilator driving mechanisms

Flow generators
   Generate a predetermined pattern of flow
   Pattern is maintained despite changes in compliance and airway resistance

   Advantages:
   ● Maintain tidal volume in absence of leaks

   Disadvantages:
   ● Decrease in compliance increases peak alveolar pressure and may cause barotrauma

Pressure generators
   Generate a relatively low pressure
   Resulting flow pattern affected by resistance and compliance

   Advantages:
   ● Control of peak airway and alveolar pressure minimises risk of barotrauma
   ● Maintain tidal volume despite variable, small leaks
   ● Maximum tidal volume for given airway pressure
   ● Early filling of lung may improve gas exchange

   Disadvantages:
   ● Tidal volume affected by changed impedances

increased alveolar pressure is adequate to expel the inspired volume within the available expiratory time, but flow will still be continuing at the end of each phase of respiration. The resulting "intrinsic" PEEP (also called "alveolar" or "auto" PEEP) will increase mean intrathoracic pressure and so tend to reduce cardiac output.

In clinical practice an increase in airway resistance is often accompanied by a decrease in compliance, so that the time constant of the whole lung is reduced towards normal. However, if compliance is decreased without any change in resistance the time constant is decreased, so that filling is completed rapidly but tidal volume is also decreased (fig 3.3). In the pressure generation mode, tidal volume is affected not only by the airway pressure and compliance, but also by the airway resistance and duration of inspiration. Continuous monitoring of expired volume is therefore essential. However, a pressure generator has two major advantages. Firstly, the inflation pressure cannot exceed the set value. This reduces the risk of barotrauma and enables the tracheal cuff pressure to be maintained at a minimal level. Secondly, a pressure generator tends to maintain a constant tidal volume despite small variable leaks in the circuit. It is therefore particularly useful in neonates and children, where it is customary to use a loose fitting uncuffed tube, and in adults, where prolonged use of a cuff tube has resulted in tracheal dilatation and difficulty in maintaining an airtight connection with the trachea.

In the earlier mechanical ventilators the design of the driving mechanism determined whether it behaved as a flow generator or pressure generator. For example, in the Cape and Engström ventilators the use of a mechanical linkage between a powerful electric motor and a bellows or piston ensured that the gas left the driving mechanism with a repeatable flow pattern; these machines could be classified as flow generators. On the other hand, in the Radcliffe and Barnet ventilators a bellows was compressed by weights or a spring – this mechanism resulted in a ventilator which had the characteristics of a pressure generator.

The basic characteristic could be modified by other features. For example, if there was a pressure limiting valve in the breathing system of a flow generator, the ventilator would function as a flow generator while the airway pressure was below the limiting pressure but as a pressure generator after the limiting pressure had been exceeded. The presence of a large compliance, such as a humidifier, in the breathing system also tended to downgrade the flow generator characteristics. Similarly, if a pressure generator was set to develop a high pressure and then caused to discharge through a high internal resistance it might behave as a flow generator because any changes in resistance in the patient would be small in comparison with the internal resistance of the ventilator.

In most modern machines increased flexibility has been provided by controlling the flow from a high pressure gas source with rapidly acting inspiratory and expiratory valves. By using feedback control from flow or pressure sensors in the breathing system, the machine can function either as a flow generator or a pressure generator, depending on the setting of the controls. However, if the distinction between the two modes of gas delivery is kept in mind, much confusion will be avoided.

Flow and pressure generators: expiratory phase. Since expiration is usually passive, expiratory flow will depend on the alveolar pressure generated by the tidal volume and lung compliance and on the resistance of the expiratory pathway. Since the alveolar pressure decreases approximately exponentially as the lung empties, expiratory flow also decays exponentially. Most ventilators may, therefore, be classified as pressure generators during expiration. However, if the pattern of expiratory flow were to be controlled by, say, a rapidly acting servo controlled valve, the ventilator might be classified as a flow generator in expiration. The pattern of expiratory flow may also be affected by the incorporation of a PEEP valve in the expiratory limb of the breathing system.

Cycling mechanisms

The second characteristic of ventilator function, the method of cycling from one phase to the other, is more commonly subject to operator control (table 3.1). In most machines the duration of inspiration is controlled by some sort of timing device so that the machine is time cycled.

In a volume cycled machine inspiration ceases when a preset volume has been delivered, irrespective of the time taken to achieve this. A machine that delivers a fixed flow of gas for a given time will result in the delivery of a constant tidal volume but is actually time cycled and not volume cycled. In a true volume cycled machine the cycling mechanism is tripped when a given volume has been delivered, even if the flow rate is altered by a change in respiratory impedance. In some of the newer machines the volume cycling is effected by the signal from a flow measuring device situated at the patient Y piece. With this arrangement a true volume cycled machine will compensate for a leak in the breathing system but a time cycled machine will not.

In a flow cycled machine inspiration is terminated when flow has fallen to a given level. This level may be preset or may be a proportion of the peak flow generated during inspiration.

Pressure cycling is another method of cycling which is frequently used to ensure that a preset inflation pressure is not exceeded. However, it can be used only with a flow generator or with a pressure generator that delivers an increasing pressure throughout inspiration.

In many machines several cycling mechanisms may be available. For example, in the inspiratory support mode the termination of inspiration is usually flow cycled, but pressure and time cycling mechanisms come into play if preset limits are exceeded.

Cycling from expiration to inspiration is usually time cycled when the machine is used in the controlled ventilation mode. In modern practice it is common for the inspiration to be patient cycled. Patient cycling is usually effected by sensing the small decrease in pressure in the breathing system resulting from the initiation of inspiratory flow by the patient, a sensitive trigger mechanism being activated by a reduction in pressure of 0.5–2 cm H_2O. In some machines the trigger mechanism is cycled directly by the patient's inspiratory flow. This flow cycled type of trigger can be made very sensitive but may then respond to vibrations in the breathing system or other spurious signals.

A variation of this principle is used in the flow-by system which was originally unique to the Puritan Bennett 7200 series of ventilators (see chapter 6) but is now being used in other machines. In this system a small flow of gas circulates round the breathing system during expiration and the machine is triggered when the patient's inspiration causes the flow in the expiratory tube to be less than that in the inspiratory tube. This system results in minimal delay and little increase in the work of breathing. It also seems to minimise false triggering, which is common when the breathing tubes are disturbed. This is always a problem with triggering mechanisms when the trigger sensitivity is increased towards its maximum.

Tests of ventilator performance

Few machines satisfy the above criteria completely and their performance under clinical conditions often differs considerably from the manufacturer's specification. For this reason the British and International Standards Organisations have produced recommended test procedures which are designed to reveal deficiencies in performance when the machines are stressed, as they might be in clinical practice.[7] The ventilators are connected to model lungs with adjustable compliances, and resistances and pressure, flow, and volume traces are recorded at frequencies and tidal volumes that are appropriate for the sphere of use (adult, paediatric, or neonatal) for which the ventilator was designed. In a more recent document the testing procedure has been broadened to include spontaneous breathing modes.[8] The tests not infrequently reveal unsuspected deficiencies in design that might have unfortunate clinical consequences.[9]

Ventilator design

Most ventilators consist of a mixing device, which controls the composition of the inspired gas; a driving mechanism, which forces the gas into the patient; and a breathing system, which connects the ventilator with the patient and ensures proper separation of inspired and expired gas streams. The breathing system usually incorporates some form of gas conditioning system for humidifying and, possibly, filtering the inspired gas. The ventilator will also incorporate some means of controlling positive end expiratory pressure and some monitoring devices.

Gas mixing systems

In the early ventilators the oxygen concentration was controlled by feeding oxygen into the proximal end of a reservoir tube attached to the inspiratory bellows and allowing it to flow retrogradely to the atmosphere. The oxygen was aspirated into the bellows during the refilling phase and any deficiency in volume made up by air, so that the oxygen concentration could be calculated from the oxygen flow and the delivered minute volume. In ventilators driven by compressed gas the gas mixing was effected by flow meters or by a blender attached to the pipeline supplies. In the first generation of electronic ventilators the control of oxygen concentration was accomplished by proportional mixing devices situated before the inspiratory flow control valve. In the latest generation of machines both the mixing and control of flow are effected by only two precision valves, one on the oxygen line and one on the air line. These are electronically controlled and have very rapid response times so that they can produce variable flow patterns.

Driving mechanisms

To appreciate the enormous advances in ventilator design over the past 40 years it is helpful to compare the driving mechanisms used today with some of those used in the past. In most ventilators the driving mechanism acted directly on the respired gas, but in some machines a separate source of driving gas was used to compress a flexible reservoir containing the respired gas. This facilitated sterilisation of the respired gas pathway and the control of gas concentrations but often impaired the performance of the ventilator as a flow generator, since the volume of gas between the driving source and the reservoir was compressed during inspiration and so impaired the transmission of the driving flow profile to the gas in the reservoir. The generator flow pattern was further debased by the compression of the volume of gas in the bellows and breathing system.

Flow generators. The earliest flow generators, such as the Beaver, Smith-Clarke, and Engström ventilators, used a bellows or piston connected to an approximately sinusoidal drive mechanism powered by an electric motor. With such a mechanism inspiration and expiration each occupied half of the cycle (180°). To produce a more generally acceptable inspiratory-expiratory ratio of 1:2, the Smith-Clarke and, later, Cape ventilators used mechanically controlled valves to control flow to and from the patient. The inspiratory valve opened after the bellows had completed 60° of the cycle and

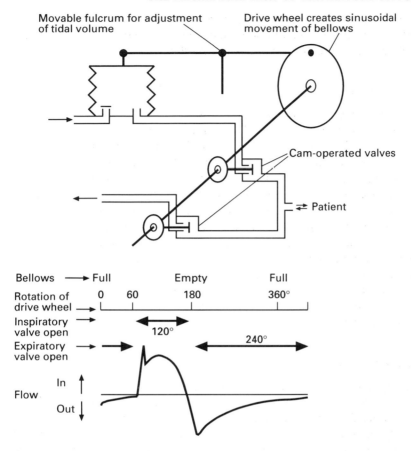

Fig 3.4 Method of achieving I:E ratio of 1:2 with sine wave driving mechanism in Smith-Clarke and Cape ventilators. Inspiratory valve was not opened until bellows had completed one third of its stroke; expiratory valve remained open during this period. In Smith-Clarke ventilator, high initial flow of compressed gas from bellows was buffered by large volume humidifier.

expiration was prolonged by allowing expiratory gas flow during this period (fig 3.4). This system caused the ventilator to function transiently as a pressure generator as the gas compressed in the bellows was discharged into the patient, but it then became a flow generator for the remainder of inspiration. The Engström used a piston to compress the reservoir bag of the breathing system and achieved a similar inspiratory-expiratory ratio by spilling gas from the piston during the later part of inspiration (fig 3.5).

In the American Emerson ventilator, which also used a large piston and cylinder, the inspiratory-expiratory ratio was controlled by varying the speed of the electric motor during inspiration and expiration.

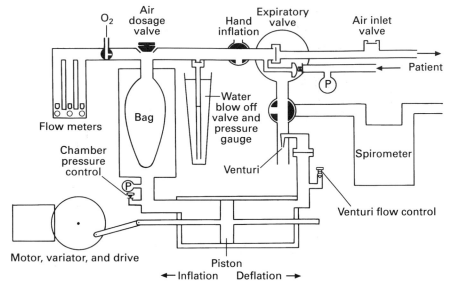

Fig 3.5 Engström 200 ventilator. The large piston was driven by an electric motor. During expiration it generated negative pressure around the bag; this aspirated air into the bag through the calibrated dosage valve. This could be supplemented by oxygen or replaced by other gases supplied by flow meters. On the return stroke the piston compressed gas around the bag, rate of inspiratory flow being determined by an adjustable valve which controlled chamber pressure. The piston could also be used to activate the venturi, which provided negative pressure during expiration.

Providing that the motor was powerful enough to drive the bellows or piston in the predetermined pattern, such systems should have acted as perfect flow generators. In most of the early ventilators, however, such perfection was never attained because of the presence of a large compressed gas volume or internal compliance. There were two sources of inefficiency (fig 3.6). Firstly, a proportion of the gas issuing from the bellows was compressed in the ventilator tubes and humidifier and so did not reach the lungs. With rigid delivery tubes the loss of delivered volume was proportional to the internal volume of the tubes and humidifier and could be calculated from Boyle's law. If corrugated rubber tubes were used there was an additional volume loss due to the increase in their internal volume with increased inflation pressure. Under the worst conditions the volume loss might amount to 400–500 ml at an inflation pressure of 50 cm H_2O.[10] This volume of gas re-expanded on expiration so that a spirometer placed in the expiratory limb of the breathing system would overestimate the volume delivered to the lung.

The second source of inefficiency was the volume of gas left in the bellows at the end of each stroke. This caused the delivered volume to be less than that predicted from the displacement of the bellows. This was a particular

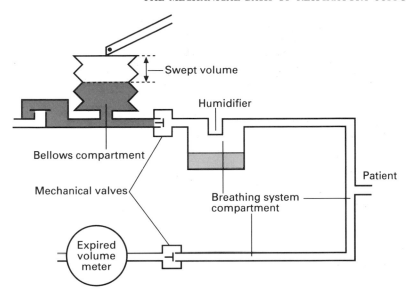

Fig 3.6 Sources of internal compliance. Volume of gas delivered by bellows is less than swept volume because a proportion of this gas is compressed within bellows compartment. Gas compressed in tubing and humidifier is also not delivered to patient but re-expands on expiration and is recorded by expired volume meter.

problem in Blease ventilators where the tidal volume was indicated by a calibrated scale on the transparent cylinder surrounding the hanging second stage bellows. The error was greatest when small tidal volumes were used and residual volume was large, and decreased when the bellows was more completely emptied by the delivery of large tidal volumes. The residual volume in the bellows in most other ventilators was minimised by emptying the bellows completely at the end of each inspiration whatever the stroke volume. In modern ventilators using a second stage system (for example, the Engström Elvira) care is taken to minimise the volume in the flexible reservoir and breathing system. In most machines the flow pattern is maintained by monitoring the delivered flow profile and then using servocontrol of the inspiratory valve to ensure that the flow pattern is maintained within predetermined limits. However, in a ventilator such as the Siemens Servo 900 the driving pressure in the pressurised bellows supplying the inspiratory valve is generally set to a relatively low level (about 60 cm H_2O) so that the flow profile may not be maintained if the impedances to inflation are high. In the newer ventilators higher driving pressures are used so that the flow profile is less affected by changes in the lungs. Furthermore, the availability of low volume humidifiers and non-elastic tubing ensures that the internal compliance of the breathing system in modern ventilators does not exceed 0.2–0.3 l kPa^{-1} (2–3 ml/cm H_2O).

In a number of older machines, such as the Bennett MA1, the gas flow was generated by a fan or blower and the duration of inspiration and expiration controlled by mechanical valves which intermittently connected the source of pressure to the lungs. Unfortunately, most fan or blower units are sensitive to back pressure so that flow decreased as the pressure in the airways increased. Such machines thus showed many of the characteristics of a pressure generator, with flow and tidal volume decreasing as airway pressure increased. This problem could have been overcome by using a high pressure gas source connected in series with a high resistance so that back pressure had a minimal effect. However, with the technology available at the time it would have been difficult to produce variable tidal volumes and flow patterns with such a system.

Pressure generators. Because of fears that airway pressures above 3 kPa (30 cm H_2O) might cause lung damage, most of the early flow generators were fitted with safety valves to prevent high pressures reaching the patient, and it was because of these fears that pressure generators or pressure cycled machines were widely used in the early days of mechanical ventilation. The pressure was generated either by a weight or a spring acting on a bellows. One of the earliest pressure generators was the Radcliffe ventilator. This was based on the Oxford inflating bellows, which was pressurised by weights added to the upper end of the bellows. The bellows was expanded by a simple fork lift mechanism which raised the upper end during expiration and then released it to produce inspiration. The pressure was constant throughout inspiration and was adjusted by altering the number of weights. The inspiratory-expiratory ratio was fixed at 1:2 and the frequency could be changed in steps by the use of a simple bicycle gearbox. The ventilator was initially used with a pressure operated non-rebreathing valve close to the patient. This tended to stick when wet, and the later East-Radcliffe machines were fitted with cam operated mechanical valves.

Other machines, such as the Barnet ventilator, used compressed gas from a compressor or pipeline to inflate a bellows against the pressure exerted by a spring. Electronically timed valves were then used to control the gas flow to and from the patient. The Barnet was one of the first ventilators to permit inspiratory and expiratory times to be adjusted independently. Tidal volume was determined by the volume of fresh gas fed into the bellows and by the respiratory frequency, so the machine could also be classified as a minute volume divider. Because the pressure exerted by the spring decreased somewhat as the bellows emptied, this behaved as a decreasing pressure generator. As a consequence, flow decreased more rapidly during inspiration than with the square wave of pressure produced by the Radcliffe ventilator. It was also necessary to ensure that the spring tension was adequate to drive the gas into the patient during the set inspiratory time.

Another ventilator which functioned as a pressure generator and minute

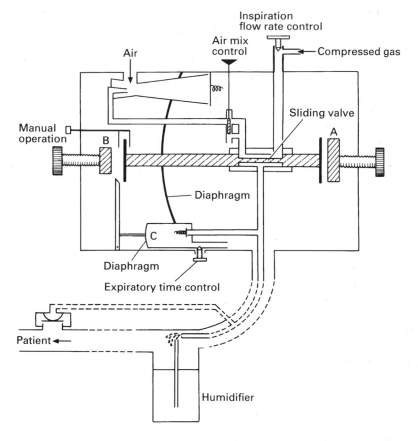

Fig 3.7 Principle of earlier designs of Bird ventilator.

volume divider was the Manley.[11] In this machine a controlled flow of fresh gas was fed into a weighted bellows and the expiratory time adjusted by a valve mechanically linked to a timing bellows. Modified versions of this ventilator are still widely used during anaesthesia.

One other way of overcoming the problems associated with high pressure was to use pressure cycling. This approach was characterised by the Bird series of ventilators and by the Bennett PR2. In the Bird series (fig 3.7) a constant flow of gas from a high pressure source (4 atmospheres) was directed into the patient through a nebuliser and non-rebreathing valve, the expiratory diaphragm of the latter being closed during inspiration by pressure from the fresh gas line. The fresh gas flow was controlled by a sliding valve which was held in the inspiratory position by a magnet (A). The valve was also attached to a diaphragm which formed one wall of the main chamber of the ventilator. As the pressure in the patient and chamber built up during

69

inspiration, a point was reached where the pressure on the diaphragm overcame the attraction of magnet (A) so that the valve flipped into the expiratory position, thus terminating fresh gas flow and allowing the expiratory valve at the patient to open. The pressure at which this occurred depended on the position of magnet (A). Expiration was terminated by the lever which separated the valve rod from magnet (B). Since this level was connected to the diaphragm at the end of chamber (C), it moved to the left when the chamber was pressurised during inspiration and moved to the right when the chamber was decompressed at a controlled rate by the variable leak during separation. It was possible to adjust the position of magnet (B) so that a small drop in pressure in the main chamber flipped the diaphragm into the inspiratory position, thus enabling the machine to be patient-triggered.

The machine could be classified as a flow generator with pressure cycling from inspiration to expiration, but time cycling or patient cycling from expiration to inspiration. When only the driving gas (oxygen) was being delivered to the patient the ventilator behaved as a flow generator. However, there was also a venturi air-mix device which could be used to dilute the driving gas, and this was affected by back pressure so that flow through it decreased during inspiration. This caused the oxygen concentration to increase as the airway pressure increased and degraded the flow generator characteristics.

Design of modern ventilators

Pneumatic system

Although there is, as yet, little firm evidence that using any of the newer ventilatory modes has any effect on mortality, manufacturers have been forced to produce ventilators capable of generating them. This needed completely new design concepts.

The first generation of such machines was electronically controlled and was typified by the Siemens Servo 900 series. The inspired gas is provided by pipelines, mixed by calibrated blenders, and collected in a reservoir which is pressurised to about 60 cm H_2O. Flow from this reservoir is then controlled by altering the aperture of a rapidly acting inspiratory valve. The inspiratory flow rate is measured continuously by a flow meter placed just after the inspiratory valve, and the valve is then servocontrolled to produce the desired flow pattern, inspiratory time, and tidal volume. This system enables the ventilator to adjust the resistance of the inspiratory valve to maintain a preset flow pattern despite changes in the patient's lungs. A second valve on the expiratory side can be used to control expiratory time and flow and can be linked to the airway pressure so that it can be used to maintain a given level of PEEP (fig 3.8).

This system provides great flexibility and enables the ventilator to be

---

Changes in ventilator design

Early designs

Advantages:
- One driving mechanism: function easily understood
- Few controls, monitors limited to pressure and expired volume
- Robust and relatively cheap
- Few required pressurised gas sources
- Some could be operated by hand in event of power failure
- Some had facility for autoclaving all the gas pathway
- Could usually be maintained by relatively unskilled staff

Disadvantages:
- Usually only one driving mechanism
- Flow pattern distorted by large internal compliance or lack of power
- Mechanical patient-triggering: delay and lack of sensitivity
- No spontaneous breathing modes other than assisted ventilation

Modern designs

Advantages:
- One machine can generate most modern ventilatory modes
- Can be updated by changing software
- Sophisticated monitoring and alarm systems
- Sensitive and rapid response patient-triggering systems

Disadvantages:
- Expensive
- Require electric power and pressurised gas sources
- Large number of controls and complex monitoring systems
- High incidence of false alarms
- Require skilled maintenance

---

converted into a pressure generator by reducing the spring pressure on the reservoir bellows and opening the inspiratory valve so that flow is determined by the pressure and the characteristics of the patient's lungs. The electronic control units enable the ventilator to calculate the appropriate inspiratory flow required to produce a given tidal volume in a given inspiratory time with any pattern of flow, and it is easy to incorporate an inspiratory pause or to synchronise a mandatory breath with the patient's spontaneous respiration. The machine achieves safety by imposing limits on a number of the controls and by adjustable alarm limits on the expired volume and airway pressure monitors.

The second generation of machines uses more advanced microprocessor technology. This has enabled additional modes to be added, and it provides the possibility of adding new modes simply by importing new software. Additional modes require more controls and more sophisticated monitoring (for example, to separate the patient's spontaneous breathing component

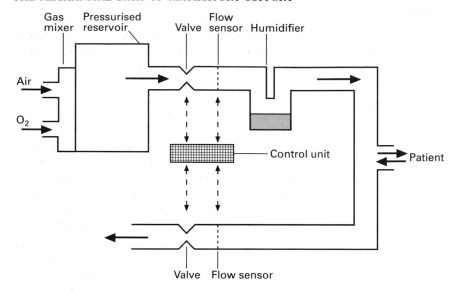

Fig 3.8 Basic design of Servo 900 series of ventilators.

from the machine component during mandatory minute volume ventilation), and this has resulted in a much more complicated machine which could easily be programmed incorrectly by the operator. To guard against improper settings manufacturers have therefore had to add more monitors and complicated alarm systems. Many of the controls are rarely used, and this makes the machine expensive and much less attractive to medical and nursing staff.

The breathing system

Although concentric tube breathing systems have been used for some paediatric and adult ventilators they are not in general use. A concentric tube system had the advantage that the inspired gas contained in the inner tube could be warmed by the expired gas in the outer tube, but resistance considerations resulted in a larger than normal diameter of outer tube, which was cumbersome in use. There were also problems with the connections. Double tube systems are therefore now almost universal.

The tubing should be transparent, have a low resistance, and be flexible and it should not be expanded significantly by the increased internal pressure. Humidifiers should have a small internal volume and low resistance. They should be capable of delivering fully saturated gas at 37 °C to the patient without condensation of water vapour in the inspiratory tube, and there should be provision for the drainage of the water vapour that condenses in the expiratory tube. Heat and moisture exchangers and bacterial filters should have a low internal volume and resistance, and the filters should not be affected by moisture or secretions. Connections should be capable of being locked in position to prevent accidental disconnection.

Devices used for generating positive end expiratory pressure

A positive end expiratory pressure can be generated during controlled mechanical ventilation and continuous positive airway pressure breathing in several ways (fig 3.9), but many of these fail to achieve the ideal characteristics – those of a threshold resistor, where the airway pressure is kept constant throughout a wide range of flows. The least satisfactory is a constriction in the expiratory line. This functions as an orifice so that the pressure difference across the resistance is proportional to the square of flow rate. Such an arrangement results in maximal retardation of flow at the beginning of expiration, when flow is at a peak, and so holds the intrathoracic pressure at a higher level than necessary throughout expiration. The small orifice required to create the resistance is easily blocked, and the patient will generate a very high airway pressure if the flow rate is suddenly increased by coughing. This method is no longer used.

A very safe method of producing PEEP is to pass the expired gas through a wide tube (at least 2 cm in diameter) dipping under water. There is an additional impedance to flow at the beginning of expiration due to the inertia of the water column which is displaced from the tube, but the system acts as a threshold resistor when flow is established. A valve in which PEEP is created by a column of water or a weight acting on a diaphragm has similar characteristics. Most PEEP valves now use a spring loaded diaphragm. Many of the earlier designs had marked flow dependency because they were designed with a short spring, which exerted a progressively higher pressure as the diaphragm was lifted off its seating by the higher flows. However, most of the spring loaded valves now in use have relatively long, or specially designed, springs to ensure that the pressure remains constant over a wide range of flows. PEEP may also be generated by using a jet to create a retrograde flow of gas into the expiratory pathway.

Modern ventilators providing a CPAP or PEEP mode overcome these problems by electronic control of inspiratory and expiratory flow. The inspiratory valve opens when the pressure in the breathing system is decreased by the patient's inspiration and then adjusts the flow to provide the preset CPAP level throughout inspiration. When the patient starts to breathe out, the inspiratory valve closes and the expiratory valve opens. As the pressure in the airway falls the expiratory valve progressively closes, so maintaining the desired level of CPAP or PEEP with minimal restriction of expiratory flow.

73

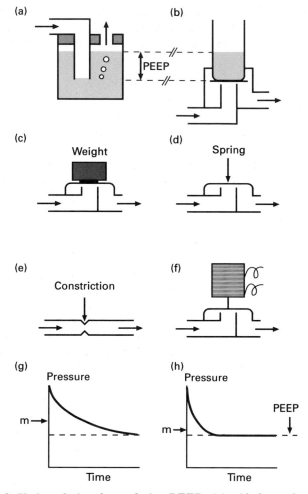

Fig 3.9 (a-f) Various devices for producing PEEP: (a) wide bore tube dipping under water; (b) non-return valve weighted by column of water; (c) non-return valve with adjustable weight; (d) non-return valve pressurised by spring; (e) constriction in expiratory pathway; (f) electromagnetically controlled valve in ventilator. (g) Airway pressure during expiration using device (e); (h) pressure trace using device (f). Note higher mean airway pressure (m) in (g) than (h).

Monitoring devices

All ventilators should be fitted with a device for measuring airway pressure and with an expired volume meter. These should have adjustable high and low alarm limits. Pressure and volume should ideally be measured at the patient Y piece, but moisture and dead space limitations increase the technical difficulties. The problem of malfunction due to moisture and

74

secretions can be reduced by placing a heat and moisture exchanger between the device and patient, but this increases dead space and resistance. For these reasons measurements of pressure and volume are usually made within the machine.

Measuring pressure. Many machines incorporate an aneroid gauge for measuring pressure. Such gauges are remarkably robust and rarely need recalibration. However, their speed of response is limited and it is difficult to detect rapid changes in pressure by watching the movement of the pointer.

Most modern ventilators now use electronic pressure measurement devices. These produce analogue signals which enable dynamic traces to be displayed. The traces can also be analysed for the digital display of such variables as peak, inspiratory pause, and mean or end expiratory pressure. These pressures can then be used for the on line calculation of respiratory mechanics (p 33).

Measuring flow. In most modern ventilators volume is derived from electronic integration of the flow signal, though some use separate devices for measuring flow and volume. The standard device for measuring flow is the pneumotachograph. This consists of a sensitive differential transducer which measures the difference in pressure across a resistance element (fig 3.10). In the original Fleisch pneumotachograph the resistor consisted of a bundle of parallel sided tubes which were heated to prevent water condensation affecting the resistance. Flow through these tubes was laminar, so that the pressure difference was directly proportional to flow rate. In the Lilly type of head a wire mesh was used as the laminar resistance element. In both these devices some of the air passages could become blocked by secretions, with a consequent alteration in resistance. The difference in gas composition and temperature between inspired and expired gas must also be taken into account when calibrating the system.

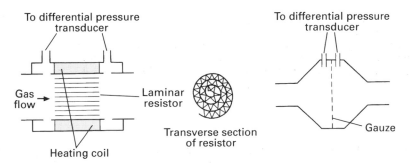

Fig 3.10 (left; centre) Longitudinal and transverse sections of a Fleisch pneumotachograph head. The resistance unit is made by winding corrugated foil into a spiral, so creating a series of parallel sided tubes. These are heated to prevent condensation. (right) Lilly type head with wire mesh resistance element.

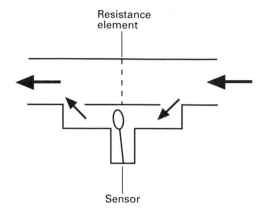

Fig 3.11 Flowmeter system used in Servo 900 series of ventilators. Wire mesh resistance element causes proportion of flow to be directed through smaller tube, where it produces deflection of small disc attached to lever. Deflection is measured by strain gauge which provides electrical signal proportional to flow.

The flow meters in the Siemens Servo 900 series ventilators use a modified pneumotachograph system for measuring flow (fig 3.11). The main stream of gas passes through a gauze resistor; a small proportion is directed through a bypass tube and its flow is measured by the displacement of a small disc attached to a lever and electronic sensing unit. The entry to the expiratory measuring system is sloped upwards to discourage the flow of water into the system, and the whole assembly is heated to prevent condensation. The flow meter must be calibrated at regular intervals.

Most of the problems associated with pneumotachographs have now been overcome by the development of a new head that uses a variable orifice as the

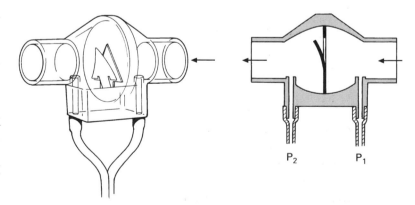

Fig 3.12 Variable orifice, variable pressure drop flow transducer. V shaped flap ensures that pressure drop across orifice is directly proportional to flow rate.

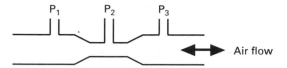

Fig 3.13 Bidirectional venturi flowmeter. Pressure at P_2 is less than pressure at P_1 or P_3.

resistance component (fig 3.12). The resistance element consists of a diaphragm with a hinged, V shaped flap in its centre and pressure tappings on either side of the diaphragm. The pressure drop across an orifice is normally related to the square of flow rate, but in this device the size of orifice

---

Devices used to measure flow

Pneumotachograph used in:
  Siemens Servo 900 series
  Hamilton Veolar

Venturi flowmeter used in:
  Engström Elvira

Hot wire flowmeter used in:
  Dräger Evita
  Puritan Bennett 7200 series

Devices used to measure expired volume

Dry gas meter:
  Smith-Clarke
  Engström 200, 300 series

Wright respirometer:
  Cape
  East-Radcliffe

Dräger volumeter:
  Early Dräger ventilators

Bellows in perspex chamber:
  Bennett MA1

Bag in rigid chamber:
  Engström Elvira

Integration of expired flow signal:
  Other modern ventilators

77

increases with flow so that a linear relation between flow and pressure difference is maintained. The head has a small dead space and is light, disposable, and not affected by moisture. It represents a remarkable technological achievement and is used to measure flow at the Y piece with the Hamilton Veolar ventilator. The development of very sensitive, stable, differential pressure transducers has now opened the way for the introduction of even simpler flow measuring devices – with microprocessor technology, non-linear signals can be linearised with ease. Thus the drop in pressure along a tube can be used as a measure of flow.

Another device used to measure flow is the venturi-type flowmeter (fig 3.13). This uses a differential transducer to sense the difference in lateral pressure created by the difference in gas velocity between the wide and narrow parts of the tube, the lateral pressure being least in regions where velocity is highest. This form of sensor is used to measure inspiratory flow in the Engström Elvira ventilator. There is a 6% difference in reading between air and oxygen, but this can be corrected by the microprocessor as the composition of the inspired gas is known.

The other commonly used flow meter is the hot wire device. This measures the rate of heat loss from a hot wire. The heat loss depends on the flow and the thermal conductivity of the gas, and therefore depends on gas composition, but with modern technology it is easy to incorporate correction factors which enable accurate readings to be obtained. Hot wire flow meters are used in the Dräger Evita and Puritan Bennett 7200 series ventilators.

Measuring expired volume. In the earlier ventilators expired volume was measured by a dry gas meter[12] or one of the more portable devices such as the Wright respirometer or Dräger volumeter. The Wright respirometer consists of a light mica vane which is rotated by directing the expired gas through a series of slits in a cylinder that surrounds the vane. The rate of rotation is related to the flow rate, and the flow rate can be integrated mechanically or electronically. The device is affected by the composition of the gas and by the pattern of flow and tends to over-read at high flows and under-read at low flows. Its accuracy is also affected by the condensation of water within the casing. The Dräger device is a true volume meter and is therefore not affected by the characteristics of the gas. It consists of two interlocking rotors which segregate a known volume of gas during each revolution, so that the volume is directly related to the number of revolutions of the rotors.

There are other true expired volume monitors. In the Bennett MA1 machine the expired gas was directed into a lightweight bellows, the volume being read from the excursion of the bellows within a perspex cylinder. The bellows was then emptied during the next inspiration. The Engström Elvira uses a unique method of measuring expired volume, which is also not affected by gas composition. The expired gas is directed into a bag situated within a rigid chamber. During the next inspiration the bag is compressed by a known flow of gas into the chamber and the expired volume calculated from the time taken to empty the bag.

Gas analysis. Inspired oxygen is usually measured with a polarographic sensor or galvanic cell. Rapid paramagnetic analysers are used to measure breath by breath differences between inspired and expired oxygen concentrations in some metabolic computers.[12]

Other monitoring. In modern machines the microprocessor is used to process data from the ventilator control module and the flow, pressure, and volume sensors to provide other information of value to the operator. For example, it is now possible to display spontaneous breathing rate and spontaneous minute volume separately from the ventilator delivered volume. This may then be used to control the level of support when using the mandatory minute volume mode. However, the choice of monitoring display depends on the design of the ventilator. For example, reference to table 6.2 shows that most modern ventilators require the setting of four main controls to determine the rate, depth, and pattern of each controlled breath. The settings of these controls determine the value of a fifth variable, which may be peak flow, inspiratory pause time, or inspiratory-expiratory ratio. Peak flow is of little importance, so it is not displayed on the Siemens Servo 900. On the other hand, inspiratory-expiratory ratio is important, so the Puritan Bennett 7200 provides an alarm to warn the operator if this is outside the normal range.

Sterilisation

In the 1960s ventilators were sterilised before use by circulating ethylene oxide or formaldehyde vapour around the circuit. This procedure was time consuming and carried the risk of contamination of the inspired gas by residual agent leaching out of the circuit components. Later ventilators such as the Oxford, Cape Bristol, and Engström 300 had breathing systems that could be removed and autoclaved (fig 3.14). Most ventilators now permit disposal or sterilisation of the breathing system components and expiratory valve units; others rely on the use of disposable bacterial filters to separate the patient from the ventilator.

Conclusions

The modern ventilator uses precision mechanical components and microprocessor technology to generate a wide variety of ventilatory modes. This provides great flexibility and allows manufacturers to incorporate new modes by adding new software. However, the addition of extra modes increases the time required to set up each machine for use and adds to the complexity of

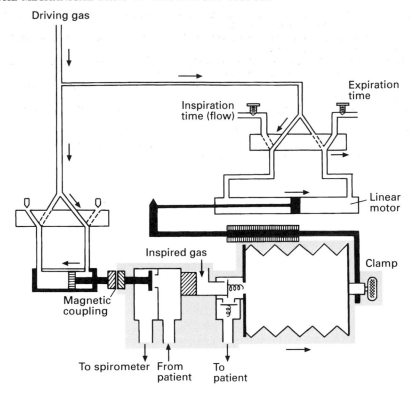

Fig 3.14 Oxford ventilator: a constant flow, time cycled ventilator with detachable bellows and valve unit (stippled area) that can be sterilised by autoclaving. The arrows show the direction of movement during expiration. The components within the shaded area can be removed for autoclaving.

both the controls and the monitoring system. Such machines do not necessarily increase the quality of patient care. Those inexperienced in the use of such machines should choose one or two simple modes (such as controlled mechanical ventilation or synchronised intermittent mandatory ventilation – see chapter 4) and master their use before embarking on the use of other modes. If in doubt use a simple ventilator with controlled ventilation: it will probably do less harm in the long term!

1 Mushin WW, Rendell-Baker L, Thompson PW, Mapleson WW. *Automatic ventilation of the lungs*. 3rd ed. Oxford: Blackwell Scientific, 1980.
2 Kirby RR, Banner MJ, Downs JB. *Clinical applications of ventilatory support*. Edinburgh: Churchill Livingstone, 1990.
3 Tobin MJ. *Principles and practice of mechanical ventilation*. New York: McGraw-Hill, 1994.
4 Bersten AD, Skowronski GA, Oh TE. New generation ventilators. *Anaesth Intensive Care* 1986;**14**:293–305.
5 Smallwood RW. Ventilators-reported classifications and their usefulness. *Anaesth Intensive Care* 1986;**14**:251–7.

6 Mapleson WW. The effects of changes of lung characteristics on the functioning of automatic ventilators. *Anaesthesia* 1962;**17**:300–14.

7 International Organization for Standardization. *ISO 5369. Breathing machines for medical use—lung ventilators.* Geneva: ISO, 1987.

8 British Standards Organisation. *BS 5724. Medical Electrical Equipment, Part 3. Particular requirements for performance.* London: BSO, Section 3. 1991:12.

9 Loh L, Sykes MK, Chakrabarti MK. The assessment of ventilator performance. *Br J Anaesth* 1978;**50**:63–71.

10 Loh L, Chakrabarti MK. The internal compliance of ventilators. *Anaesthesia* 1971;**26**:414–20.

11 Manley RW. A new mechanical ventilator. *Anaesthesia* 1961;**16**:317–25.

12 Sykes MK, Vickers MD, Hull CJ. *Principles of measurement and monitoring in anaesthesia and intensive care.* 3rd ed. Oxford: Blackwell Scientific, 1991.

4 Respiratory support: techniques for reducing mean airway pressure

During the first two decades after the introduction of long term intermittent positive pressure ventilation most units in Scandinavia and the United Kingdom used ventilators that controlled ventilation at a fixed frequency. In the United States and some other parts of Europe it was more common to use patient triggered (assisted) ventilation in patients who had normal respiratory control mechanisms. The difference in practice was partly due to the fact that North American anaesthetists had been using small doses of a muscle relaxant with manual assistance to ventilation during anaesthesia, whereas the British had always used larger doses of relaxant with controlled ventilation, but it was also influenced by the availability of the Bennett and Bird intermittent positive pressure breathing machines, which had been developed in the United States in the early 1950s.

By the early seventies it had become apparent that the addition of a positive end expiratory pressure during controlled mechanical ventilation was an effective method of increasing arterial PO_2 in patients with severe acute lung disease.[1] It was soon recognised, however, that the resulting high mean intrathoracic pressures often produced a decrease in cardiac output, which caused the oxygen delivery to the tissues to be reduced instead of increased.[2] It was also realised that the high peak airway pressures resulting from the addition of a positive end expiratory pressure were causing an increased incidence of barotrauma. These problems initially led to an interest in techniques that could minimise mean intrathoracic pressure by allowing the patient to breathe spontaneously for all or part of the time, and subsequently to techniques that were primarily designed to reduce peak airway pressure. This chapter will deal with the various spontaneous breathing modes that are designed to reduce mean intrathoracic pressure, and the next chapter will consider the problem of barotrauma and techniques designed to decrease peak airway pressure.

Techniques that minimise the increase in mean intrathoracic pressure

Patients with acute lung disease invariably have a defect in oxygen transfer due to the presence of ventilation-perfusion inequalities or an increase in intrapulmonary shunt. These changes may or may not be accompanied by CO_2 retention. The increase in shunt is usually due to pneumonic consolidation or to alveolar collapse. Collapse may be due to bronchial blockage by secretions or to alveolar flooding in severe pulmonary oedema. Both consolidation and collapse reduce the number of ventilated alveoli and so result in a decrease in lung compliance and functional residual capacity. If the functional residual capacity is increased by the application of a positive end expiratory pressure (PEEP), a proportion of the collapsed alveoli may be re-expanded, thus decreasing the shunt and increasing the arterial PO_2. In patients who are capable of breathing spontaneously, the increase in end expiratory lung volume can be achieved by connecting the patient to a continuous positive airway pressure breathing system. However, if the patient already has an increased PCO_2, or hypoventilates when treated with CPAP, it will be necessary to add some form of ventilatory support to ensure adequate CO_2 elimination.

Spontaneous breathing without ventilatory support

Continuous positive airway pressure breathing (CPAP, CPPB) was first used in the 1930s for treating asthma and pulmonary oedema by Barach in the United States[3] and by Poulton in the United Kingdom.[4] It was, however, only used sporadically until the 1970s, when it was advocated for the treatment of respiratory distress in neonates and adults.[5, 6]

The positive airway pressure is applied by connecting the patient to a breathing system that can generate a constant pressure up to levels of 2 kPa (20 cm H_2O) above atmospheric. If the patient is conscious and cooperative, and treatment is likely to be required for a matter of hours, the connection to the breathing system can be effected by the use of a tightly fitting face mask held in place by a head harness. With such a system it may be necessary to pass a nasogastric tube to prevent gastric distension, though this tends to impair the fit of the mask. For longer applications a tracheal tube or tracheostomy is required. CPAP is now also used for the treatment of obstructive sleep apnoea and may then be administered by nasal prongs or a nasal mask. Nasal prongs work particularly well in neonates requiring CPAP since they are obligatory nose breathers.[7] In neonates and small children lung volume may also be increased by exposing the trunk to a constant subatmospheric pressure by means of a body box fitted with a neck seal.[8]

CPAP: requirements

There are two essentials for the successful application of CPAP. The first is that there should be no rebreathing. The second is that there should be minimal variation in the airway pressure (less than 1–2 cm H_2O) throughout

83

the respiratory cycle, for any decrease in airway pressure during inspiration, or increase during expiration, will increase the work of breathing.[9]

CPAP systems are basically of two types – those using a continuous flow of fresh gas and those providing an intermittent flow during inspiration. The former exist as independent systems for they do not require any of the mechanical or electronic devices associated with a ventilator, but the latter must be incorporated into a ventilator since they rely on the ventilator's monitoring and control mechanisms. Both systems are capable of fulfilling the requirements enumerated above. However, they can be used successfully only if their basic principles are thoroughly understood. For this reason the factors governing rebreathing in the various breathing systems used in anaesthesia and intensive care will be considered first and their use in CPAP systems then discussed.

Continuous flow breathing systems

CO_2 absorption systems. Circle or to-and-fro CO_2 absorption systems are frequently used during anaesthesia (fig 4.1). However, the absorber is bulky, the absorbent requires frequent replacement, and there is a danger of inhaling irritant soda lime dust. Such systems are, therefore, rarely used in intensive care units.

Non-rebreathing system. An equally effective method of eliminating CO_2 is to use a non-rebreathing valve system (fig 4.1). In this system the fresh gas is stored in a reservoir bag and inspired via the wide bore delivery tube and inspiratory valve. During expiration the inspiratory valve closes and the expiratory valve opens so that the expired gas passes out to atmosphere. Since all the expired gas is eliminated from the system, fresh gas flow must exceed the minute volume. The inspiratory and expiratory valves are usually placed close to the patient to minimise mixing of inspired and expired gas, but in this position they are liable to malfunction because of condensation of water vapour, so other breathing systems are more commonly used.

Other systems. These systems have been classified and subjected to theoretical analysis by Mapleson.[10] The systems most commonly used in intensive care are the Mapleson A, D, and E (fig 4.2). The common feature of all these systems is that standard wide bore tubing (with an internal volume exceeding the tidal volume) is used to maintain the separation of fresh gas, dead space gas, and alveolar gas before the alveolar gas is washed out of the system. In the A system the reservoir bag and reservoir tube constitute the afferent limb of the system, whereas in the D and E systems the reservoir is situated in the efferent limb. These differences have a major effect on CO_2 elimination.

In the Mapleson A system, at the end of inspiration the reservoir bag is partially deflated while the expiratory valve is closed by the light pressure

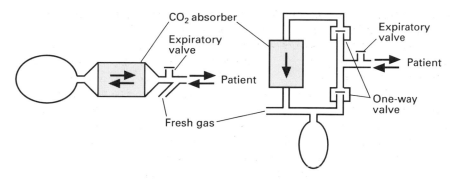

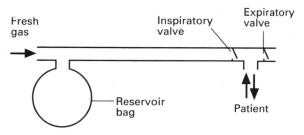

Fig 4.1 CO₂ absorption and non-rebreathing systems. (top left) To and fro absorption system (Waters cannister). Absorption cannister is sometimes removed when system is used for emergency resuscitation. It then functions as a Mapleson C system and requires a fresh gas flow equal to three times the minute volume to ensure adequate CO₂ elimination. (top right) Circle absorption system. (bottom) Non-rebreathing system with inspiratory and expiratory valves.

exerted by the spring. During expiration the dead space gas (approximately 150 ml) and the alveolar gas (approximately 350 ml) flow retrogradely into the tube connecting the reservoir bag to the patient (fig 4.2). The internal volume of this tube must be greater than two thirds of the tidal volume, so that alveolar gas does not enter the reservoir bag and contaminate the fresh gas. Towards the end of expiration fresh gas overflows from the reservoir bag and drives the expired gas back down the tube and out through the expiratory valve. The dead space gas is approximately one third of the tidal volume and, since it contains no CO_2, it may be re-inhaled without affecting CO_2 clearance. Rebreathing is therefore prevented by supplying a fresh gas flow which is at least two thirds of the minute volume. In practice, the fresh gas flow is usually set to exceed the minute volume to allow for variations in ventilation and dead space.

Although the expiratory valve is normally mounted close to the patient, it

85

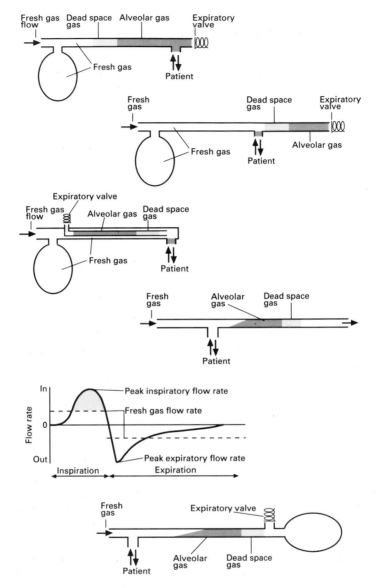

Fig 4.2 Spontaneous breathing systems: (top left) Mapleson A system: mid-expiration just before opening of expiratory valve; (top right) T piece modification of Mapleson A system at end expiration; (centre left) Lack version of Mapleson A system at end expiration; (centre right) Mapleson E system at end expiration; (bottom left) pattern of gas flow during a spontaneous breath. Peak inspiratory flow rate is usually $2\frac{1}{2}$ times minute volume, but varies with the inspiratory flow pattern. Shaded area shows flow that will be re-inhaled from expiratory limb of E system if fresh gas flow rate is less than inspiratory flow rate; (bottom right) Mapleson D has similar characteristics to E system – reservoir bag and expiratory valve at outlet from expiratory tube facilitate manual ventilation.

Continuous flow breathing systems

System	Fresh gas flow requirement

CO_2 absorption:
  To and fro
  Circle
	>Patient's oxygen consumption

Non-rebreathing	>Patient's minute volume

Mapleson classification:
  A (single tube)
  A (Lack version)
  A (T-piece version)
	>$\frac{2}{3}$ patient's minute volume

D E	>2–3 times patient's minute volume

may be separated from the patient by a length of wide bore tubing. This tubing may form the expiratory limb of a T piece arrangement or may be mounted concentrically, as in the Lack version of the Mapleson A system (fig 4.2). With the latter arrangement, the expiratory valve is mounted close to the reservoir bag so that it can be easily adjusted should manual assistance to ventilation be required during anaesthesia. Neither of these variations affects the behaviour of the system and fresh gas flow requirements are similar to the standard Mapleson A system.

The Mapleson E system is based on the T piece arrangement. The patient receives a continuous flow of fresh gas from the inspiratory tube (which can be narrow bore since it does not receive respired gas), and both fresh gas and expired gas accumulate in the expiratory tube during expiration. The patient's expiratory flow rate is maximal at the beginning of expiration, so there is little dilution of dead space gas and alveolar gas with fresh gas. As expiration proceeds the flow rate declines exponentially, so that there is a progressively increasing concentration of fresh gas in the expiratory tube. More fresh gas flows into the expiratory tube during the expiratory pause. If the fresh gas flow rate exceeds the peak inspiratory flow rate (usually $2\frac{1}{2}$–3 times the minute volume), no gas will be reinhaled from this tube. However, if the fresh gas flow is less than the peak inspiratory flow rate, the balance will be provided by gas from the expiratory tube (fig 4.2). The composition of the gas that is reinhaled will depend on the relation between the fresh gas flow rate and the inspiratory and expiratory flow patterns, but it is usually recommended that the fresh gas flow rate should exceed 2–3 times the minute volume to eliminate the possibility of rebreathing alveolar gas.

The Mapleson D version of the T piece system has a reservoir bag and expiratory valve at the outlet from the expiratory tube to facilitate manual ventilation (fig 4.2). As the reservoir is on the efferent limb, this has similar characteristics to the E system.

Clinical CPAP systems

A CPAP system for clinical use requires a source of fresh gas, an oxygen analyser to monitor its composition, and a valve to generate the positive pressure. If the patient is intubated, it will also be necessary to provide a means of humidifying the inspired gas.

Continuous flow systems. The two continuous flow breathing systems used for administering CPAP are based on the Mapleson systems described above. The high flow system (fig 4.3) is based on the Mapleson E system and so requires a fresh gas flow rate that exceeds the patient's peak inspiratory flow rate (normally two to three times the minute volume) to prevent rebreathing. Since patients with respiratory distress often have peak inspiratory flow rates of more than 60 l/min, it is necessary to supply fresh gas at a flow rate of 60–80 l/min to minimise the decrease in circuit pressure during inspiration. This is accomplished most economically by using an oxygen driven injector to entrain ambient air, but with all injector systems it is important to ensure that the delivered flow rate and oxygen concentration are not affected by the back pressure in the breathing system. The high flow system is simple to use but requires a very efficient humidifier to warm and moisten the high flow of fresh gas. It also requires a PEEP device that can tolerate high expiratory flows without increasing the CPAP pressure.

The low flow system incorporates a reservoir in the inspiratory limb (fig 4.3). This must be used with a PEEP device that incorporates a one way expiratory valve. It then behaves as a Mapleson A system, so that rebreathing is prevented by a fresh gas flow rate that exceeds the patient's minute

---

Clinical CPAP systems

System	Fresh gas flow requirement
Continuous flow systems:	
High flow, no reservoir	>Peak inspiratory flow rate (30–80 l/min)
Low flow, proximal reservoir	>Patient's minute volume
Low flow, distal reservoir	>2–3 times patient's minute volume
Demand valve systems	= Patient's minute volume
Nasal CPAP	>50 l/min

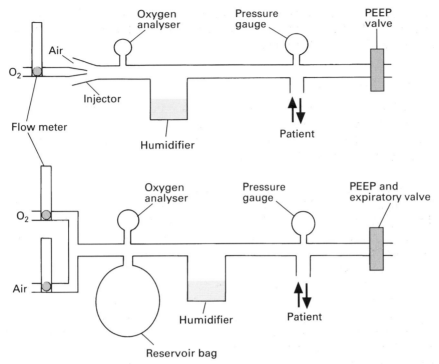

Fig 4.3 Continuous flow CPAP systems. (top) High flow system without reservoir. PEEP valve prevents reinhalation from expiratory limb, so fresh gas flow must exceed peak inspiratory flow rate. (bottom) Low flow system with reservoir. This functions as Mapleson A system.

volume.[10] In this system gas from the reservoir supplements the continuous fresh gas flow during inspiration, the reservoir being refilled during expiration.

The reservoir must be capable of maintaining a constant pressure during inspiration in order to prevent any decrease in circuit pressure during this phase. There are two ways of ensuring this. One is to modify the reservoir bag so that it delivers the tidal volume with a small change in pressure. This can be accomplished by using either a very distensible bag (which has a high compliance) or very large bag (so that the tidal volume constitutes a very small proportion of the total volume). A very large bag occupies a great deal of space; it has been found that the best compromise is provided by a thin-walled 5–10 l latex bag which has a compliance of 5–10 l kPa^{-1} (0.5–1 l/cm H_2O) throughout the range of pressures used. Some commercial CPAP systems achieve acceptable control of the inspiratory pressure by using a moderately compliant bag with a 30–40 l/min flow of fresh gas, thus striking a compromise between the high and low flow systems.

The second method of stabilising the inspiratory pressure is to use a

89

weighted bellows as the reservoir.[11] If this bellows is on the inspiratory limb the breathing system will have the characteristics of the Mapleson A system so that rebreathing will not occur if the fresh gas flow exceeds the patient's minute volume, but if the bag is placed on the expiratory limb the system will behave as a Mapleson D system (fig 4.4). This requires a fresh gas flow of at least three times the minute volume to prevent rebreathing. Both of these systems enable the difference between inspired and expired pressures to be maintained at less than 1–2 cm H_2O, providing the other components of the circuit are of the appropriate standard.

Obviously, the resistance of the tubes and connections to the patient must be reduced to the minimum. The resistance of the humidifier is not critical with the T piece system because the gas is driven through it by the high pressure source, but it is of great importance when the reservoir system is placed upstream from the humidifier, since flow through the humidifier is then generated by the patient. Hot water humidifiers used with a reservoir system should have a resistance of less than 1–2 cm H_2O at a flow rate of 60 l/min and should be capable of providing adequate humidity at this flow rate.

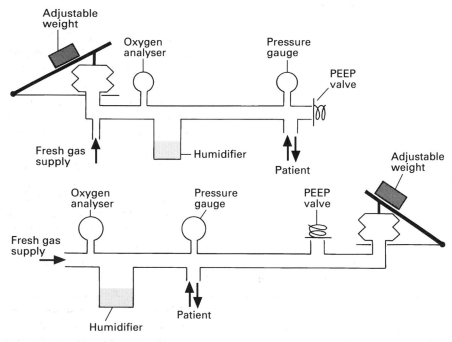

Fig 4.4 Use of weighted bellows to maintain constant pressure during inspiration and expiration. (top) Mapleson A system; (bottom) Mapleson D system. The Mapleson A system requires fresh gas flow approximately equal to minute volume; the D system requires flow equal to three times minute volume.

Criteria for CPAP systems

General
- Pressure at patient connection must not vary by more than 1–2 cm H_2O
- Fresh gas flow must be adequate to clear CO_2 from system
- System pressure must not increase by more than 1–2 cm H_2O when expiratory flow is increased by coughing

With demand valve systems
- Patient trigger mechanism must respond to small changes in pressure or flow
- Must have short response time
- Ventilator must generate sufficient flow to satisfy patient demand

---

The remaining component that governs the variation in pressure within the system is the device used to generate the positive pressure. The characteristics of this device are of crucial importance and need to approximate to those of a threshold resistor – that is, the pressure difference across the valve should not vary with flow.[12] The various devices used for this purpose have been described in chapter 3.

Demand valve systems. Many modern ventilators provide a CPAP mode. The inspiratory valve on the ventilator is opened when the triggering mechanism is activated by the patient's inspiration, and the flow through the valve is then continuously adjusted to maintain the set pressure during inspiration. The expiratory phase is triggered by a decrease in inspiratory flow rate or by a transient increase in pressure in the breathing system when the patient exhales, and the expiratory valve then controls the expiratory flow rate to maintain the desired CPAP level during expiration. Although it is very convenient to have the CPAP system integrated with the ventilator, it must be recognised that the work of breathing is usually higher with a demand system than with a continuous flow system. There are two reasons for this: the patient has to trigger the inspiration, and some ventilators are unable to provide the high peak inspiratory flows required by patients in respiratory failure. The efficiency of a ventilator CPAP system depends, therefore, on the efficiency of the triggering system, the design of the gas delivery module, and the speed of response of the servosystem controlling the valves.

In the older ventilators the patient triggering mechanisms were usually activated by a decrease in pressure in the ventilator or breathing system, but since they were based on mechanical components they were relatively insensitive and slow to respond. Modern systems use electronic pressure sensors and valves and so have greater sensitivity and speed of response. However, there are still large variations between machines.[13] Although most trigger mechanisms are activated by a decrease in pressure in the breathing system, some (Engström Elvira and Hamilton Veolar, for example) are triggered by inspiratory flow. Another system, which has deservedly become very popular, is the so called flow-by system used in the Puritan Bennett 7200 series of ventilators. This utilises a low, constant flow of gas which is circulated round the breathing system, triggering being effected by the decrease in flow in the expiratory limb when the patient inspires. This type of trigger has a very short response time and minimises the work of breathing required to initiate inspiration.[13] [14] With some ventilators it is now possible to measure the airway pressure at the patient Y piece and to use this pressure to trigger the machine. This can also contribute to a reduction in the work of breathing.[15]

The second characteristic, the ability of the ventilator to follow the patient's ventilatory pattern, depends on the accuracy and speed of response of the servosystem controlling the valves and on the design of the gas delivery system. Patients in respiratory failure often generate high peak flows early in inspiration, so it may be necessary for the ventilator to deliver a flow of 50–100 l/min shortly after the inspiratory valve opens.[16] Some ventilators cannot meet this demand.[17] Although measurements of the inspiratory work of breathing show that work is minimal when the patient breathes from a well designed continuous flow CPAP breathing system, demand valve systems are now much improved, and some ventilators now approach this ideal.[18]

The patient also has to overcome the resistance of the tracheal tube and ventilator breathing system. Hot water humidifiers in which the inspired gas passes over the surface of the water or over a wick usually create little resistance to gas flow, but in those in which the gas bubbles through water (for example, the Bennett Cascade) the resistance is much greater. This type of humidifier should never be used with spontaneous breathing modes, for the patient has to generate a large subatmospheric pressure to overcome the resistance imposed by the water, and this both delays the triggering of the ventilator and increases the work of breathing. Since other components, such as bacterial filters and heat and moisture exchangers, may double the work imposed by the tracheal tube resistance,[19] it is important to check the breathing system's resistance before using the system with a spontaneously breathing patient. These components may also increase the apparatus dead space and so impose an extra load on spontaneously breathing patients.

Other CPAP systems. Nasal CPAP is now frequently used in the domiciliary setting to treat obstructive sleep apnoea. The pressures required are in the range 0.5–1 kPa (5–10 cm H_2O) and there is usually no requirement for extra oxygen. To meet this demand high capacity blower units have been developed. These units provide a high flow of air which is directed across a T piece through an expiratory orifice with a diameter of 2 mm. The blower acts as a pressure generator and the flow through the orifice is considerably higher than the patient's inspiratory flow rate, so the pressure at the nose is reasonably well maintained throughout both phases of respiration. Such units are portable, quiet, and reliable and provide a relatively cheap method of administering nocturnal CPAP (see pp 236–7).

Monitoring

As the inspired oxygen concentration may be reduced by failure of the oxygen supply, leaks in the oxygen line, or the effects of back pressure on the oxygen flowmeter, the oxygen blender, or the injector, the inspired concentration should be monitored continuously. The airway pressure should be sensed as close to the tracheal tube as possible and displayed continuously. Pulse oximetry provides a useful guide to the efficiency of treatment. As the high gas flow rates make measuring the expired volume difficult, end tidal CO_2 monitoring or regular blood gas measurements will be required to detect the onset of hypoventilation.

Indications for CPAP

CPAP is often administered by nasal mask to maintain upper airway patency in patients who have episodes of obstructive apnoea during sleep. It may also be administered by face mask or tracheal tube as the first line of treatment in conditions such as pneumonia, pulmonary oedema, and atelectasis, in which an increase in end expiratory lung volume may be expected to improve oxygenation. CPAP has been used in many other situations.[20] It has proved of value during weaning from mechanical ventilation and has been used to splint the chest wall in patients with a flail chest, to improve lung function in patients with diaphragmatic paralysis, and to reduce the frequency of apnoeic attacks in premature infants.

CPAP often increases arterial saturation and may, in some circumstances, decrease the work of breathing by moving the tidal volume onto a steeper part of the pressure-volume curve.[21] The lower levels of CPAP may improve the distribution of ventilation and so reduce dead space to tidal volume ratio and shunt; higher levels may compress the pulmonary capillaries and so increase dead space and decrease cardiac output. Careful monitoring of the blood gases and circulation is therefore required.

Spontaneous breathing with ventilatory assistance

Although the use of CPAP may maintain adequate oxygenation during the most critical phase of acute lung disease, in many patients the increased work of breathing or depression of respiratory drive produced by hypoxia, sepsis, or other factors will lead to hypoventilation. It is then necessary to consider other modes which incorporate some form of ventilatory assistance. Two techniques that improve CO_2 elimination by periodically reducing the level of

CPAP (airway pressure release ventilation and biphasic positive pressure ventilation) were originally designed to reduce peak airway pressure and are therefore discussed in the next chapter. The remainder (box; fig 4.5) are discussed below.

Assisted mechanical ventilation (AMV)

When a ventilator is set to provide controlled ventilation the machine delivers a breath at regular intervals, the frequency and pattern of the breath being determined by the ventilator controls and by the characteristics of the machine. (If the machine is being used in the pressure generation mode, the breath pattern will also depend on the mechanical characteristics of the respiratory system.) When the machine is set to provide assisted ventilation and the trigger sensitivity is correctly adjusted, the machine delivers a breath with each spontaneous inspiration, so that the patient can control the total ventilation by altering the frequency of breathing (fig 4.5). In addition, some ventilators have an assist/control mode in which the ventilator will deliver a mandatory breath if the machine has not been patient triggered within a given time interval.

This apparently simple concept never proved popular in the United Kingdom, for patients often "fought the ventilator." The failure to achieve

---

Ventilatory modes that reduce mean intrathoracic pressure

Ventilatory mode	Assistance to ventilation
Continuous positive airway pressure breathing	Nil
Airway pressure release ventilation	Intermittent lung deflation for 1–2 seconds
Biphasic positive airway pressure	Alternating high and low CPAP
Intermittent mandatory ventilation	Mandatory breath at intervals
Synchronised intermittent mandatory ventilation	Mandatory breaths synchronised with some spontaneous breaths
Mandatory minute volume	Addition of mandatory breaths or inspiratory pressure support until preset minute volume achieved
Assisted mechanical ventilation	All mandatory breaths patient triggered
Inspiratory pressure support	Pressure support with each patient triggered breath

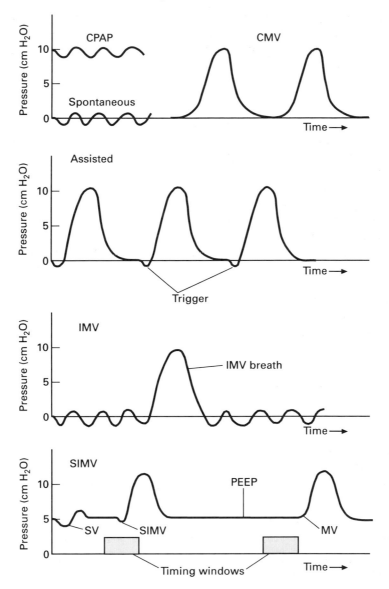

Fig 4.5 Airway pressure traces with various breathing modes. (top left) Continuous positive airway pressure breathing (CPAP), spontaneous breathing, and controlled mechanical ventilation (CMV); (top right) assisted ventilation, showing subatmospheric triggering pressure; (bottom left) intermittent mandatory ventilation, showing IMV breath superimposed on spontaneous breathing; (bottom right) synchronised intermittent mandatory ventilation showing spontaneous breath (SV) followed by synchronised mandatory breath (SIMV). As no spontaneous breath occurred during second timing window, ventilator delivered mandatory breath (MV) at preset interval. System is pressurised to PEEP of 5 cm H$_2$O.

synchronisation with the ventilator was probably due to several causes. Firstly, the early trigger mechanisms were relatively insensitive and required a decrease in airway pressure of 1–2 cm H_2O to activate them. Secondly, there was an appreciable time delay between the beginning of the patient's spontaneous inspiration and the delivery of the machine breath. The third possible cause of patient discomfort was the fixed pattern of the machine breath; this was often very different from the patient's spontaneous breathing pattern and so failed to relieve the patient of the inspiratory work of breathing. Indeed, it has been shown that most patients continue to inspire actively during an assisted breath and so expend 30–50% of the energy required for a passive expansion to the same lung volume.[22]

Intermittent mandatory ventilation (IMV)

With the assist mode and inspiratory pressure support, the assistance is provided with each triggered breath. Other modes permit the patient to breathe spontaneously and only provide a mandatory breath at intervals. The first technique to be introduced was intermittent mandatory ventilation (IMV).[23] The patient breathes spontaneously through a breathing system which provides humidified gases with the appropriate concentration of oxygen, and the machine then delivers a mandatory breath of predetermined characteristics at preset intervals (fig 4.5).

Originally, two breathing systems linked by a non-return valve were used (fig 4.6). The patient breathed spontaneously from a continuous high or low flow CPAP system with expiratory valve, and this was then isolated from the ventilator breathing system by the closure of the non-return valve when the pressure in the inspiratory limb was increased by the delivery of a mandatory breath.

The use of two breathing systems was cumbersome and increased the risks of leaks and disconnections. Furthermore, it was necessary to ensure that the spontaneous breathing system fulfilled all the criteria for an efficient CPAP system and that the inspired oxygen was matched to that in the ventilator. Another difficulty was that monitoring of expired minute volume was precluded by the continuous gas flow through the CPAP system. These difficulties have been largely overcome in modern ventilators, which provide both spontaneous and mandatory breaths with a single breathing system (fig 4.6). However, the characteristics of the various machines vary widely and it is important to ensure that the work of breathing during the spontaneous breaths is not increased by an insensitive trigger mechanism or an inadequate inspiratory flow capability.[24]

The main disadvantage of IMV is that the mandatory breath is not synchronised with the patient's inspiration so that "stacking" of the mandatory breath on top of the spontaneous breath can occur. This may lead to a high peak airway pressure. The technique was originally introduced to

96

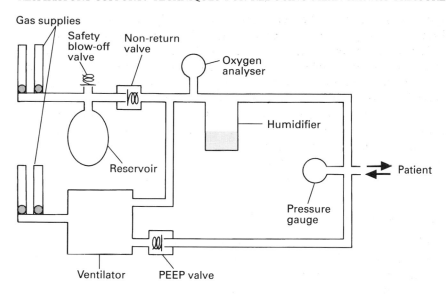

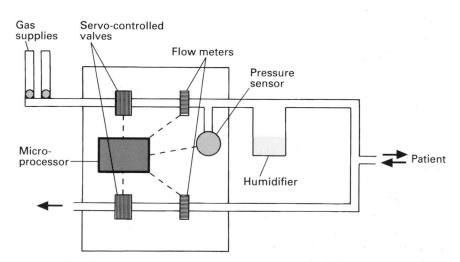

Fig 4.6 Intermittent mandatory ventilation (IMV) breathing systems. (top) Separate spontaneous breathing and ventilator systems. (bottom) Ventilator combined system.

facilitate weaning, the idea being that the frequency of the mandatory breaths could be gradually reduced (for example, to 4 bpm) as the patient's spontaneous efforts improved. However, in many units, the technique is often utilised for the whole duration of treatment when patients do not have a primary disorder of respiratory control.[25] As with the other spontaneous

97

breathing techniques, the appropriate degree of end expiratory pressure can be applied during both spontaneous and mandatory breaths by incorporating a PEEP valve in the expiratory limb of the breathing system.

Synchronised intermittent mandatory ventilation (SIMV)

The next development, which was designed to prevent the "stacking" of breaths, was synchronised intermittent mandatory ventilation. This mode was incorporated in the Siemens Servo ventilator, which was introduced in the early 1970s, and enabled the mandatory breath to be synchronised with a spontaneous breath. To allow the patient to take spontaneous breaths between the mandatory breaths, the machine creates a regular time window which is the only period during which the ventilator will trigger in response to a spontaneous breath (fig 4.5). The duration and frequency of this window is usually controlled by the mandatory and SIMV frequency controls, the duration of the window being determined by the mandatory frequency control, and the frequency of its occurrence being adjusted by the SIMV frequency control. For example, if the mandatory breath frequency is set to 15 bpm and the SIMV frequency to 6 bpm, the duration of the window is $60 \div 15 = 4$ seconds, and the maximum interval between the mandatory breaths is $60 \div 6 = 10$ seconds. The patient is thus able to breath spontaneously without triggering the ventilator for 6 seconds, but any spontaneous breath occurring in the next 4 seconds will trigger a mandatory breath. If no spontaneous breath is detected during this 4 second period, the ventilator will then deliver a mandatory breath. The completely apnoeic patient thus receives six mandatory breaths per minute.

The main problem with SIMV is that the mandatory breath rate may not provide adequate ventilation if the patient becomes apnoeic and so fails to trigger synchronised breaths. Careful monitoring of respiratory rate is therefore required. Although SIMV would be expected to reduce the peak inspiratory pressure resulting from the stacking of breaths during the delivery of a mandatory breath, there is little evidence that it has any other advantages over IMV. Studies in critically ill patients, and in anaesthetised dogs subjected to near drowning, showed that although peak inspiratory pressures were higher during IMV than SIMV, there were no significant differences in cardiovascular variables or shunt.[26, 27] One explanation might be that patients on IMV usually learn to synchronise their breathing pattern with the IMV rate.

Mandatory minute volume (MMV)

A third technique that combines spontaneous breathing with mandatory breaths from the ventilator is mandatory minute volume. This is a mode that tailors the patient's minute volume to the value which the physician considers to be appropriate for the patient.[28] In the original system this volume of gas was fed into the bellows of a ventilator and the patient was then allowed to breathe from the bellows. If the patient's minute volume fell below the mandatory minute volume the gas accumulated in the bellows. When the bellows expanded beyond a certain point an inspiration was triggered so that the patient received a mandatory breath to make up for the deficiency in spontaneous breathing. The MMV mode is attractive in theory, but it is of limited practical value because it is difficult to judge what minute volume the patient requires, and the ventilatory requirement may change rapidly if the patient is conscious. If the mandatory volume is inadequate the patient's respiratory rate will increase and tidal volume will tend to decrease. This leads to an increase in the ratio of dead space to tidal volume and ventilation becomes less efficient. This, in turn, produces a further increase in breathing frequency, thus creating a vicious circle.

Some modern ventilators incorporate MMV modes that are claimed to be an improvement on the original concept. For example, in the Engström Elvira the microprocessor measures the expired minute volume and durations of apnoea over a 30 second period and compares the expired volume with that set on the ventilator. If the expired volume is less than the preset value it delivers the preset tidal volume. If the patient has apnoeic periods, a time limitation function comes into play and also provides a mandatory breath. In the CPU 1 ventilator a different algorithm is used, the minute volume being maintained by adjusting the period between mandatory breaths by altering the expiration time. The Hamilton Veolar utilises yet another principle, the level of tidal volume being averaged over eight breaths and the ventilator then providing the level of inspiratory pressure support required to bring the tidal volume back to the preset level. If apnoea occurs the ventilator switches to the IMV mode.

Sophisticated monitoring techniques are required to separate the spontaneous breathing component from that delivered by the ventilator, and trend data are particularly helpful for following the patient's progress. Alarm systems are also required to warn of a reduction in spontaneous tidal volume or an increase in respiratory frequency. It has also been suggested that the monitoring of end tidal CO_2 may be used to detect problems with MMV. In the Engström Elvira, controlled ventilation is automatically resumed if the respiratory rate exceeds a preset value. The patient may also be supplied with more volume than that set on the MMV control should demand exceed the supply. Despite the theoretical attraction of the technique, there is as yet no evidence that it is superior to any of the other spontaneous breathing modes.[29]

Inspiratory pressure support (IPS)

This is one of the most important modes to be introduced in recent years and is now being widely used. In this mode the ventilator is patient triggered by each breath and the machine then provides a positive pressure throughout inspiration. In most ventilators the applied pressure is constant, but in some the pressure increases during inspiration. The pressure may be set at a low level (2–10 cm H_2O) to help the patient overcome the resistance of the breathing system, tracheal tube, and connections, or it may be set to a higher level so that it virtually abolishes the work of breathing.

The important difference between the original assist mode and inspiratory pressure support is that with the assist mode the breath pattern was fixed by the characteristics of the lung and the machine, whereas during inspiratory support it is the level of support and the patient's respiratory muscle activity which determine the flow pattern, inspiratory flow usually being terminated by the ventilator when flow decreases to about 25% of the peak flow. In most ventilators, additional safety is provided by mechanisms that terminate inspiration if it is unusually prolonged or if the peak airway pressure exceeds a preset value.[30]

The application of IPS increases tidal volume and slows respiratory rate. The technique has two important theoretical advantages over other spontaneous breathing modes. Firstly, if the patient has normal respiratory control mechanisms and the correct level of support is provided, IPS should enable the patient to adjust the ventilation to match the metabolic demand, while the oxygen cost of breathing is reduced to normal levels. Secondly, it should enable the respiratory muscles to be exercised in the normal manner, so preventing disuse atrophy and reducing weaning difficulties. Unfortunately, it is not known what level of support must be provided to achieve these aims. There are also some technical considerations associated with the generation of the applied pressure.[31]

Technical considerations. The first technical problem is the design of the patient trigger mechanism. Since the successful use of the technique depends on applying pressure support throughout the period of inspiration, it is important that the trigger mechanism should be sensitive to small changes of pressure or flow and that the ventilator should respond without delay.[13, 18]

The second technical factor to be considered is the rate at which the

---

Technical considerations in inspiratory pressure support

- Patient triggering mechanism must be sensitive and have rapid response
- Breathing system must be pressurised at appropriate rate
- Termination of inspiration usually triggered by preset decrease in flow
- Must be secondary mechanisms (time, pressure) to terminate inspiratory flow
- Respiratory rate (and, possibly, sternomastoid muscle activity) is best guide to appropriate level of support

breathing system is pressurised. A fast rate results in the application of a square wave of pressure, which might tend to inhibit further inspiratory muscle activity; a slow rate results in a more gradual build up of pressure within the system and might increase the work performed by the patient. Initial flows below or above the optimum result in faster breathing frequencies, shorter inspiratory times, and smaller tidal volumes. In general the optimal initial flow rates are highest in patients with a low compliance or a strong respiratory drive.[32] In some ventilators (Siemens Servo 900c, Dräger Evita) this flow rate can be adjusted.

The third technical consideration is the mechanism terminating inspiration. Most ventilators cycle to expiration when the flow falls to a fixed percentage (12–25%) of the peak flow, or to an absolute level of flow (2–6 l/min). Two additional mechanisms are usually provided for safety. One cycles the machine to expiration when the airway pressure is more than 2–3 cm H_2O above the IPS pressure, and the other terminates inspiration after a preset time – an essential safeguard against a possible leak from the system.

Mode of use. As the work of breathing is increased in patients with areas of collapse and a low lung volume, the first step in setting up the ventilator in the IPS mode is to set an appropriate level of PEEP so that gas exchange and respiratory mechanics are optimised (see p 206). The appropriate level of pressure support must then be chosen after considering, firstly, the work required to overcome the resistances imposed by the ventilator, breathing system, and tracheal tube or tracheostomy, and, secondly, the increased work of breathing associated with the disease process.

The resistance to breathing through the tubes and connectors of a standard breathing system with a well designed hot water humidifier or heat and moisture exchanger should not exceed 2–3 cm H_2O at a flow rate of 30 l/min. However, the addition of some heat and moisture exchangers (particularly if they include bacterial filters) may result in higher levels of resistance.[33] Furthermore, in some hot water humidifiers, such as the Bennett Cascade, the inspired gas is led under the surface of the water, thereby increasing the resistance to 3–6 cm H_2O at a flow rate of 30 l/min.

Most of the resistance encountered by the patient originates in the tracheal or tracheostomy tube and connections. This resistance is critically dependent on the geometry of tube and connections, increases non-linearly with flow rate, and is usually significantly higher than that measured in vitro since it is affected by small amounts of secretion in the tube and by the changes of shape induced by its position in the body.[34] It is also important to remember that although normal spontaneous breathing peak inspiratory flow rates are in the range 20–40 l/min, these flow rates may increase to 60–80 l/min in patients with respiratory distress. This increase in flow rate may increase the resistance of a 9 mm tracheal tube from 0.2 to 1 kPa l^{-1} s (2–10 cm $H_2O/l/s$)

and a 7 mm tube from 0.3–2.5 kPa l^{-1} s (3–25 cm $H_2O/l/s$). Studies in patients before and after extubation suggest that in most adults an IPS pressure of 8–10 cm H_2O is required to overcome the resistance of the tube and connections.[35]

The decision on the level of support to be provided to overcome the increased work of breathing resulting from the disease process is much more difficult. One suggestion is that the aim should be to supply the minimum support compatible with preventing diaphragmatic fatigue.[36] Others argue that, in the severely ill patient, the work of breathing should be reduced to normal levels in order to minimise oxygen consumption. Since too low a level will result in a high work of breathing and respiratory distress, while too high a level will result in hyperventilation and apnoea, close observation of the patient is required at all times. In general, the respiratory rate provides a good guide to the optimal level of support. If the level of support is inadequate the respiratory rate will remain raised. Adequate support should reduce the rate toward normal levels, whereas excessive support may result in a decreased rate or even in apnoeic periods. Many patients are initially treated with controlled ventilation or SIMV because the respiratory centre is depressed by residual anaesthetic or drugs used for sedation. This enables the operator to determine the airway pressure required to produce an acceptable tidal volume (approximately 10 ml/kg). When the patient is ready to be transferred to IPS the support pressure is set 3–5 cm H_2O below this and then reduced as the lung condition improves.

Another suggestion is that a high level of IPS should be used initially (25–30 cm H_2O) and that this should then be decreased in steps of 2–3 cm H_2O until palpation of the sternomastoid muscle shows phasic respiratory activity. The sternomastoid is one of the accessory muscles of respiration, and electrical activity in the muscle correlates with electromyographic signs of diaphragmatic fatigue. Since phasic contraction of the muscle indicates that diaphragmatic fatigue is present, the IPS level should then be increased by about 5 cm H_2O to relieve the load on the diaphragm.[37]

Indications. Theoretically, IPS should be the ideal mode for patients who have normal respiratory control mechanisms but inadequate ventilation. The level of PEEP can be adjusted to maintain an optimal end expiratory volume

---

Problems with inspiratory pressure support

- Inefficient patient triggering systems
- Inappropriate rate of pressurisation of system
- Difficult to decide on optimal level of support
- Requires readjustment whenever lung mechanics change

and the increase in intrathoracic pressure minimised by supplying just enough support to relieve the patient of the excessive work of breathing.

In practice, several problems limit its successful application. Firstly, there are problems associated with inefficient patient triggering systems on some ventilators and with the rate of pressurisation of the system. Secondly, there are difficulties in deciding on the optimal level of support. Thirdly, the mechanical characteristics of the patient's lungs may change rapidly, and if the patient is not being closely observed the level of support may become inadequate. Despite these difficulties inspiratory pressure support seems to be a major advance and it is now widely used during both maintenance and weaning.

Independent lung ventilation

During spontaneous ventilation in the lateral position both ventilation and blood flow are greater in the dependent than in the non-dependent lung, and ventilation and perfusion are well matched. During mechanical ventilation the distribution of blood flow is still determined by gravity but ventilation is preferentially distributed to the non-dependent lung, and ventilation-perfusion mismatch occurs. The change in the distribution of ventilation is primarily caused by the hydrostatic pressure generated by the abdominal contents, which forces the inactive diaphragm up into the chest and so reduces the dependent lung-thorax compliance and functional residual capacity. Inducing anaesthesia in the mechanically ventilated patient results in a further decrease in functional residual capacity, with the development of compression collapse in the dependent lung, so increasing intrapulmonary shunt.[38] This can be minimised by applying PEEP to the dependent lung.[39]

In patients with acute lung disease it has been shown that diffuse areas of collapse occur predominantly in the dependent areas of the lungs, and that, if the patient is rotated through 180°, these areas are redistributed to the zones of the lung now made dependent.[40] This suggests that the whole of the lung is affected by the disease process but that the weight of the oedematous lung tissue is such that it becomes impossible to ventilate the dependent lung regions with normal pressures.

One way of improving oxygenation in such patients is to rotate them at regular intervals so that the collapsed areas are moved into the non-dependent position. Blood flow in the non-dependent zones is lower than in dependent zones, so this temporarily reduces the shunt.[41] Another technique is to nurse the patient in the lateral position and apply PEEP to the dependent lung. This requires the insertion of a double lumen endobronchial tube and the separate ventilation of each lung. Since the technique is technically demanding it is usually reserved for the treatment of selected patients with severe and predominantly unilateral lung disease.

The double lumen tube should be manufactured from a tissue compatible

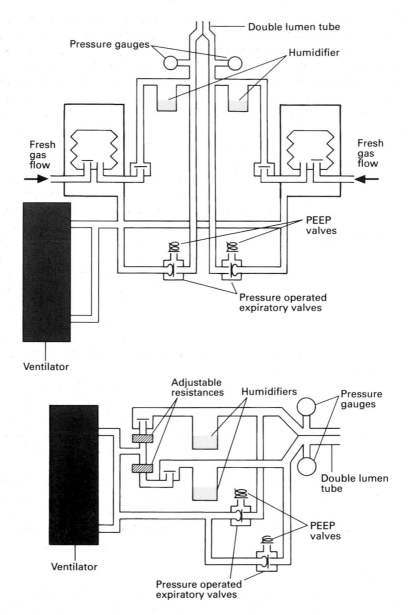

Fig 4.7 Independent lung ventilation (ILV) breathing systems. (top) Second stage bellows system. Minute volume required for ventilation of each lung is delivered into appropriate bellows from flow meters and is discharged into patient when pressure in each chamber is increased by driving ventilator. Pressure operated expiratory valves open when ventilator cycles to expiration so that expired gas can pass through PEEP valves to expired volume monitors. (bottom) Alternative system in which distribution is controlled by adjustable resistances in each inspiratory line.

plastic and have compliant cuffs. It should not have a tracheal hook, since this tends to cause ulceration of the carina. It must be of the correct size for the patient, so that the resistance is minimised. Usually a size 42 or 39 French gauge (corresponding to an internal diameter for each lumen of 6.5 and 6.0 mm) is suitable for men, and a size 37 French gauge (5.5 mm internal diameter) for women. The endobronchial limb should be inserted into the left main bronchus since this bronchus is longer than the right, the left upper lobe bronchus arising approximately 2.5 cm from the carina. Correct placement should be checked by auscultation of the upper and lower lobes during simultaneous and unilateral inflation of each lung, and by radiology and fibreoptic bronchoscopy. Cuff leakage should be checked by pressurising each tube while the other is connected to a tube dipping under water.

A double lumen tube that can be inserted through a tracheostomy is now available. This may facilitate fixation and may reduce the tube resistance. Since the bronchial cough reflex is much stronger than the tracheal cough reflex, heavy sedation or muscle paralysis is required to ensure that the tube is not displaced by coughing. It should also be remembered that the resistance of the two limbs to airflow is different and much greater than that of a single lumen tube inserted in the same patient. The increased resistance frequently results in a significant level of intrinsic PEEP which may, in itself, increase mean intrathoracic pressure and so decrease cardiac output. The presence of intrinsic PEEP is best detected by measuring airway pressures during an end expiratory pause.

Various arrangements have been described for the independent ventilation of the lungs, some using a common ventilator and some two ventilators. If a single ventilator is used some device to control the ventilation to each lung is needed. This can be either a second stage bellows that can be set to deliver a known volume,[42] or a resistor in each inspiratory line.[43] A separate PEEP valve for each lung is also needed to enable the PEEP levels to be adjusted independently (fig 4.7). The use of a single ventilator guarantees synchronisation of the ventilation to each lung but is successful only if the ventilator can generate sufficient power to overcome the various resistances to inflation. This is a particular problem if two second stage bellows are used because the volume of gas outside the bellows creates an additional compliance in the breathing system.

The use of two ventilators obviates these problems and facilitates monitoring. There was originally some concern that the lungs should be ventilated in synchrony and this required electronic linkage of the timing systems of the two ventilators.[44] It now seems that asynchronous ventilation does not compromise cardiovascular function and may permit better matching of the ventilatory parameters to the patient's lung pathology.[45]

There are no firm recommendations concerning the ventilator settings for each lung. PEEP is probably best adjusted by plotting a pressure-volume curve for each lung. This will usually show an inflexion point along the inflation limb of the curve in the diseased lung if the patient is being treated during the early stages of the disease, and the pressure at this point provides a useful guide to the initial PEEP setting (see fig 2.12). The inflation pressure in the diseased lung will inevitably be much higher than in the normal lung, but this is unlikely to lead to mediastinal displacement because the pressure will not be transmitted to the pleural space when the disease is active.

Care must be taken not to overinflate the lung when recovery occurs. Regular compliance measurements are required, independent lung ventilation being discontinued when the compliance of the diseased lung (in the supine position) increases to 60–70% of the compliance of the other lung.

Attempts have been made to apply differential PEEP in spontaneously breathing patients, but it is difficult to provide adequate sedation without depressing the respiratory control mechanisms, and the high resistance of the double lumen tube greatly increases the work of breathing.[46] High frequency jet ventilation to the damaged lung has also been combined with conventional ventilation in an attempt to reduce peak and mean pressures in patients with a bronchopleural fistula.[47]

Independent lung ventilation requires technical expertise, continuous control of the cough reflex, and careful adjustment of the ventilatory pattern delivered to each lung. Although the application of a PEEP of 10 cm H_2O to the dependent lung in patients with bilateral lung disease nursed in the lateral position has been reported to produce some improvement in gas exchange,[48] the technique seems to be of most use in patients with disease limited almost entirely to one lung. Such cases are not commonly encountered so it is not surprising that there is, as yet, no firm evidence that the technique increases survival.

Conclusions

During the past 20 years there has been rapid progress in the development of respiratory support modes that incorporate a spontaneous breathing component. Since the use of spontaneous ventilation decreases mean intra-thoracic pressure, increases the gradient for venous return, and optimises the distribution of inspired gas, it seems reasonable to allow the patient to breathe spontaneously whenever possible. In patients with lung disease, however, the pattern of spontaneous breathing may become inefficient, and this may predispose to an increase in oxygen consumption and respiratory muscle fatigue. Since there are, at present, no readily available methods of measuring respiratory muscle fatigue, the clinician must rely on observations of the frequency and pattern of breathing, together with sternomastoid muscle activity, to guide treatment.

1 Kumar A, Falke KJ, Geffin B, Aldredge CF, Laver MB, Lowenstein E, *et al.* Continuous positive-pressure ventilation in acute respiratory failure. *N Engl J Med* 1970;283:1430–6.

2 Lutch JS, Murray JF. Continuous positive-pressure ventilation: effects on systemic oxygen transport and tissue oxygenation. *Ann Intern Med* 1972;**76**:193–202.

3 Barach AL, Bickerman HA, Petty TL. Perspectives in pressure breathing. *Resp Care* 1975;**20**:627–42.

4 Poulton EP. Left-sided heart failure with pulmonary oedema. Its treatment with the "pulmonary plus pressure machine". *Lancet* 1936;**ii**:981–3.

5 Gregory GA, Kitterman JA, Phibbs RH, Tooley WH, Hamilton WK. Treatment of the idiopathic respiratory distress syndrome with continuous positive airway pressure. *N Engl J Med* 1971;**284**:1333–40.

6 Civetta JM, Brons R, Gabel JC. A simple and effective method of employing spontaneous positive pressure ventilation. Illustrative case reports. *J Thorac Cardiovasc Surg* 1972;**63**:312–7.

7 Kattwinkel J, Fleming D, Cha CC, Faranoff AA, Klaus MH. A device for administration of continuous positive airway pressure by the nasal route. *Pediatrics* 1973;**52**:131–3.

8 Chernick V, Vidyasagar D. Continuous negative chest wall pressure in hyaline membrane disease: one year experience. *Pediatrics* 1972;**49**:753–60.

9 Gherini S, Peters RM, Virgilio RW. Mechanical work on the lungs and work of breathing with positive end-expiratory pressure and continuous positive airway pressure. *Chest* 1979;**76**:251–5.

10 Mapleson WW. The elimination of rebreathing in various semiclosed anaesthetic systems. *Br J Anaesth* 1954;**26**:323–32.

11 Hillman DR, Breakey JN, Lam M, Noffsinger WJ, Finucane KE. Minimizing work of breathing with continuous positive airway pressure and intermittent mandatory ventilation: an improved continuous low-flow system. *Crit Care Med* 1987;**15**:665–70.

12 Pinsky MR, Hrehocik D, Culpepper JA, Snyder JV. Flow resistance of expiratory positive-pressure systems. *Chest* 1988;**94**:788–91.

13 Cox D, Tinloi SF, Farrimond JG. Investigation of the spontaneous modes of breathing of different ventilators. *Intensive Care Med* 1988;**14**:532–7.

14 Saito S, Tokioka H, Kosaka F. Efficacy of flow-by during continuous positive airway pressure ventilation. *Crit Care Med* 1990;**18**:654–6.

15 Banner MJ, Blanch PB, Kirby RR. Imposed work of breathing and methods of triggering a demand-flow continuous positive airway pressure system. *Crit Care Med* 1993;**21**:183–90.

16 Marini JJ, Capps JS, Culver BH. The inspiratory work of breathing during assisted mechanical ventilation. *Chest* 1985;**87**:612–8.

17 Moran JL, Homan S, O'Fatharthaigh M, Jackson M, Leppard P. Inspiratory work imposed by continuous positive airway pressure (CPAP) machines: the effect of CPAP level and endotracheal tube size. *Intensive Care Med* 1992;**18**:148–54.

18 Samodelov LF, Falke KJ. Total inspiratory work with modern demand valve devices compared to continuous flow CPAP. *Intensive Care Med* 1988;**14**:632–9.

19 Dennison FH, Taft AA, Mishoe SC, Hooker LL, Eatherly SB, Beckham RW. Analysis of resistance to gas flow in nine adult ventilator circuits. *Chest* 1989;**96**:1374–9.

20 Duncan AW, Oh TE, Hillman DR. PEEP and CPAP. *Anaesth Intensive Care* 1986;**14**:236–50.

21 Katz JA, Marks JD. Inspiratory work with and without continuous positive airway pressure in patients in acute respiratory failure. *Anesthesiology* 1985;**63**:598–607.

22 Marini JJ, Rodriguez RM, Lamb V. The inspiratory workload of patient-initiated mechanical ventilation. *Am Rev Respir Dis* 1986;**134**:902–9.

23 Downs JB, Klein EF, Desautels D, Modell JH, Kirby RR. Intermittent mandatory ventilation: a new approach to weaning patients from mechanical ventilators. *Chest* 1973;**64**:331–5.

24 Hillman K, Friedlos J, Davey A. A comparison of intermittent mandatory systems. *Crit Care Med* 1986;**14**:499–502.

25 Browne DRG, Falke K. Intermittent mandatory ventilation. In: Lemaire F, ed. *Mechanical ventilation*. 2nd ed. Berlin: Springer-Verlag, 1991.

26 Heenan TJ, Downs JB, Douglas ME, Ruiz BC, Jumper L. Intermittent mandatory ventilation: is synchronisation important? *Chest* 1980;**77**:598–602.

27 Hasten RW, Downs JB, Heenan TJ. A comparison of synchronized and non-synchronized intermittent mandatory ventilation. *Resp Care* 1980;**25**:554–7.

107

28 Hewlett AM, Platt AS, Terry VG. Mandatory minute volume: a new concept in weaning from mechanical ventilation. *Anaesthesia* 1977;**32**:163–9.
29 Laaban J-P, Ben Ayed M, Fevrier M-J. Mandatory minute volume ventilation. In: Lemaire F, ed. *Mechanical ventilation*. 2nd ed. Berlin: Springer-Verlag, 1991.
30 Brochard L, Iotti G. Pressure support ventilation. In: Lemaire F, ed. *Mechanical ventilation*. 2nd ed. Berlin: Springer-Verlag, 1991.
31 MacIntyre N, Nishimura M, Usada Y, Tokioka H, Takezawa J, Shimada Y. The Nagoya conference on system design and patient-ventilator interactions during pressure support ventilation. *Chest* 1990;**97**:1463–6.
32 MacIntyre N, Ho L. Effects of initial flow rate and breath termination criteria on pressure support ventilation. *Chest* 1991;**99**:134–8.
33 Dennison FH, Taft AA, Mishoe SC, Hooker LL, Eatherly SB, Beckham RW. Analysis of resistance to gas flow in nine adult ventilator circuits. *Chest* 1989;**96**:1374–9.
34 Wright PE, Marini JJ, Bernard GR. In vitro versus in vivo comparison of endotracheal tube airflow resistance. *Am Rev Respir Dis* 1989;**140**:10–6.
35 Fiastro JF, Habib MP, Quan SF. Pressure support compensation for inspiratory work due to endotracheal tubes and demand continuous positive airway pressure. *Chest* 1988;**93**:499–505.
36 Brochard L, Rua F, Lorino H, Lemaire F, Harf A. Inspiratory pressure support compensates for the extra work of breathing caused by the endotracheal tube. *Anesthesiology* 1991;**75**:739–45.
37 Brochard L, Harf A, Lorino H, Lemaire F. Inspiratory pressure support prevents diaphragmatic failure during weaning from mechanical ventilation. *Am Rev Respir Dis* 1989;**139**:513–21.
38 Hedenstierna G. Causes of gas exchange impairment during general anaesthesia. *Eur J Anaesthesiol* 1988;**5**:221–31.
39 Baehrendtz S, Hedenstierna G. Differential ventilation and selective positive end-expiratory pressure: effects on patients with acute bilateral lung disease. *Anesthesiology* 1984;**61**:511–7.
40 Gattinoni L, Pesenti A, Bombino M, Baglioni S, Rivolta M, Rossi G, *et al*. Relationships between lung computed tomographic density, gas exchange, and PEEP in acute respiratory failure. *Anesthesiology* 1988;**69**:824–32.
41 Langer M, Mascheroni D, Marcolin R, Gattinoni L. The prone position in ARDS patients. A clinical study. *Chest* 1988;**94**:103–7.
42 Seed RF, Sykes MK. Differential lung ventilation. *Br J Anaesth* 1972;**44**:758–66.
43 Cavanilles JM, Garrigosa F, Prieto C, Oncins JR. A selective ventilation distribution circuit (SVDC). *Intensive Care Med* 1979;**5**:95–8.
44 Carlon GC, Ray C, Klein R. Criteria for selective PEEP and independent synchronized ventilation of each lung. *Chest* 1978;**74**:501–7.
45 Hillman KM, Barber JD. Asynchronous independent lung ventilation (AILV). *Crit Care Med* 1980;**8**:390–5.
46 Crimi G, Conti G, Candiani A, Antonelli M, Bufi M, Mattia C, *et al*. Clinical use of differential continuous positive airway pressure in the treatment of unilateral acute lung injury. *Intensive Care Med* 1987;**13**:416–8.
47 Crimi G, Candiani A, Conti G, Mattia C, Gasparetto A. Clinical applications of independent lung ventilation with unilateral high frequency jet ventilation (ILV-UHFJV). *Intensive Care Med* 1986;**12**:90–4.
48 Frostell CG. Differential ventilation. *Acta Anaesthesiol Scand* 1991;**35**(Suppl.95):11.

5 Pulmonary barotrauma: techniques for reducing peak airway pressure

Causes

The problem of pulmonary barotrauma was first identified in 1827 when Leroy described how lung damage could be produced by vigorous mouth to mouth or bellows inflation of the lungs.[1] Macklin later described how the air tracked from the alveoli along the perivascular spaces to the hilum and mediastinum, where it could affect the heart and circulation.[2] Although overt barotrauma was not a problem when the use of mechanical ventilation was limited to patients with relatively normal lungs, it began to occur more frequently in the 1960s when higher airway pressures were used to treat increasing numbers of patients with severe lung disease.

In 1967 it was suggested that either high airway pressures or oxgyen toxicity might be responsible for the development of the newly recognised syndrome of bronchopulmonary dysplasia, which had been observed in neonates and adults submitted to mechanical ventilation.[3,4] Subsequent work has shown that high airway pressures may not only result in air leaks from the lung, resulting in pulmonary interstitial gas,[5] pneumothorax, pneumo-mediastinum, or subcutaneous emphysema,[6] but may also cause structural changes such as air cysts,[7] dilatation of the terminal airways,[8] or hyperinflation of a lung or lobe.[9]

It is now clear that repetitive overexpansion of the lung can lead to structural damage and oedema.[10,11] Recent experimental evidence suggests that the use of high airway pressures can also cause pulmonary capillary damage similar to that seen in the early stages of ARDS, and that the overdistension of the lung is the important factor.[12] When PEEP is applied to patients with the respiratory distress syndrome or other forms of severe lung disease there may be some recruitment of previously collapsed alveoli but most of the ventilation is directed into the relatively small areas of normal lung.[13,14] The overdistension of these areas may well result in further lung damage. For this reason there has been an increasing interest in techniques that can achieve adequate gas exchange without overdistending the normal alveoli. The techniques that will be considered are permissive hypercapnia,

---

Techniques for reducing peak airway pressure

Normal breathing frequencies
  Permissive hypercapnia
  Inverse ratio ventilation
  Continuous positive airway pressure breathing
  Airway pressure release ventilation
  Biphasic positive airway pressure ventilation

High frequency ventilation
  High frequency positive pressure ventilation
  High frequency jet ventilation
  High frequency oscillation
  High frequency chest wall oscillation

Extracorporeal gas exchange
  Extracorporeal membrane oxygenation
  Extracorporeal CO_2 removal

Intravascular gas exchange

---

inverse ratio ventilation, airway pressure release and biphasic positive pressure ventilation, continuous flow ventilation, various forms of high frequency ventilation, extracorporeal gas exchange, and the use of intravascular gas exchange devices.

Techniques using normal breathing frequencies

Permissive hypercapnia

Patients with ventilatory failure develop an increased alveolar PCO_2, which enables them to excrete the metabolic CO_2 production with a reduced minute volume. As the hypercapnia seemed to be well tolerated, Hicking and colleagues limited the peak inspiratory pressure and allowed patients with ARDS to breath spontaneously with synchronised intermittent mandatory ventilation. A retrospective analysis showed that the in hospital mortality of patients so treated was significantly lower than that predicted by a standard intensive care scoring system (Apache II).[15] Another group of patients with aspiration pneumonia treated similarly were also found on retrospective analysis to have reduced mortality.[16] These studies have not yet been confirmed by a prospective randomised trial, but they do suggest that some reduction in peak airway pressures can be achieved by allowing the arterial PCO_2 to rise to a limited extent in selected cases.[17]

Inverse ratio ventilation

It has been known for many years that prolonging the duration of inspiration decreases the ratio of physiological dead space to tidal volume and so enables more CO_2 to be eliminated with any given tidal volume.[18] Ratios of inspiratory to expiratory time (I:E) of 1:1 or 2:1 have been used to improve arterial oxygenation in neonates for many years,[19,20] the improvement in oxygenation being closely related to the increase in mean airway pressure produced by the ventilator waveform.[21] The technique has been applied to adults only during the past 15 years.

Inverse ratio ventilation (IRV) is usually tried when controlled ventilation with PEEP has failed to produce an adequate improvement in arterial oxygenation.[22] Most commonly the ventilator is set to the pressure generator mode and the inspiratory flow rate is reduced or an inspiratory hold added so that the I:E ratio is between 1:1 and 4:1. The physiological effects are variable and depend on the I:E ratio and the patient's lung disease. Prolonging the inspiratory time decreases the alveolar dead space, so that minute volume may be reduced by 10–15%. This results in a decrease in peak alveolar pressure, the peak airway pressure being further reduced by the decreased inspiratory flow rate; this results in a decreased pressure drop along the airways.

In 10 patients with acute respiratory failure due to pulmonary oedema, ARDS, or acute lung infection, a moderate prolongation of inspiration (I:E ratio 1:1 to 1.7:1) resulted in an increase in mean airway pressure and a reduction in shunt with little increase in end expiratory lung volume or decrease in cardiac output, so that oxygen delivery was increased. However, an I:E ratio of 4:1 resulted in an increase in end expiratory lung volume that varied from 465 to 2110 ml (mean 1200 ml). This was associated with an appreciable decrease in shunt, but since cardiac output was reduced by the large increase in mean airway pressure there was a decrease in oxygen delivery. In the same patients it was necessary to apply 9–19 cm H_2O PEEP (mean 13 cm H_2O) to produce similar increases in end expiratory lung volume with an inspiratory:expiratory ratio of 1:2, and this resulted in similar changes in shunt, cardiac output, and oxygen delivery.[23]

It therefore seems that ratios between 2:1 and 4:1 produce an increase in arterial PO_2 by generating intrinsic PEEP and this tends to reduce cardiac output by increasing mean intrathoracic pressure. However, ratios between 1:1 and 2:1 may decrease shunt by holding the alveoli open longer during inspiration. The main advantage of the technique over PEEP is that the reduction in dead space permits tidal volume and peak airway pressure to be reduced. However, the altered ratio and intrinsic PEEP may increase mean alveolar pressure and so decrease oxygen delivery.[24] While a moderate prolongation of inspiration may have beneficial effects on oxygen delivery and dead space, I:E ratios of more than 2:1 should be used only with careful

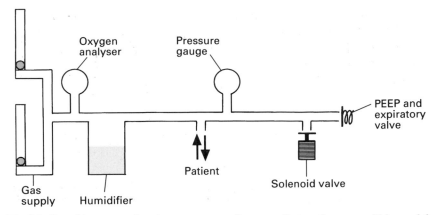

Fig 5.1 Breathing system for airway pressure release ventilation. System could be used for biphasic positive airway pressure ventilation by placing another PEEP valve in series with solenoid valve.

monitoring of the level of intrinsic PEEP and cardiovascular function, for large changes in end expiratory volume may result from small variations in regional time constants, and barotrauma may easily result.[25]

Variable airway pressure breathing

Airway pressure release ventilation and biphasic positive pressure ventilation are variants of the CPAP mode, with changes in CPAP level superimposed on spontaneous ventilation. The spontaneous breathing component decreases mean intrathoracic pressure and so reduces the effect of the high airway pressure on cardiac output. As these techniques were designed primarily to reduce peak airway pressure they are included in this chapter.

Airway pressure release ventilation (APRV). This technique was first described in 1987.[26] The patient breathes spontaneously through a high flow CPAP breathing system with an extra solenoid operated valve incorporated into the expiratory limb (fig 5.1). This valve is opened for 1–2 seconds at regular intervals so that the lung is allowed to deflate; it is then reinflated by closing the valve so that the pre-existing level of CPAP is restored. The large expiration resulting from the deflation to atmospheric pressure augments the alveolar ventilation produced by the patient's spontaneous breathing activity and so helps CO_2 excretion. Because the period during which the lung is deflated is shorter than the period of breathing at the CPAP level, the final pattern is similar to that produced by pressure-controlled inverse ratio ventilation. It differs in that the patient continues to breathe spontaneously at the CPAP level, thus minimising the intrathoracic pressure at this lung volume (fig 5.2).

112

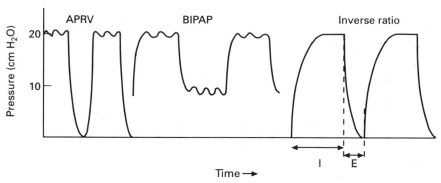

Fig 5.2 Pressure traces during airway pressure release ventilation (APRV); biphasic positive pressure ventilation (BIPAP); inverse ratio ventilation (I = inspiration, E = expiration).

The value of APRV has yet to be defined, but APRV should not be used in patients with an increased airway resistance as its success depends on a rapid emptying of the lung during the brief expiratory period. It has been suggested that it can be used as a primary mode of ventilatory support in patients who require positive end expiratory pressure with some ventilatory support. It is recommended that the CPAP level should initially be set to provide an adequate expired volume after release of the CPAP. This will depend on the compliance, so the initial CPAP level should be 10–12 cm H_2O in patients with relatively normal lungs and higher in those with reduced compliance. The frequency of deflation should be set initially to about 12 bpm and the adequacy of ventilation then assessed by observation of the patient's spontaneous breathing rate and the arterial PCO_2. It is best to aim at a frequency of deflation of less than 15 bpm. If this frequency does not provide adequate alveolar ventilation the CPAP level should be increased in increments of 2–3 cm H_2O to increase the release expired volume.

APRV has been compared with intermittent mandatory ventilation (IMV) in a group of patients with moderately severe acute lung disease. APRV provided adequate ventilation in 47 out of 50 patients.[27] Most patients were initially ventilated with intermittent mandatory ventilation using a mean peak pressure of 49 cm H_2O and an optimal level of PEEP (defined as the highest PaO_2/FiO_2 ratio without any decrease in cardiac output) of 13 cm H_2O. To achieve the same levels of PaO_2 and $PaCO_2$ on APRV, the upper pressure level had to be set to a mean of 21 cm H_2O and a positive pressure of 6 cm H_2O had to be added during the period of release, thus converting the technique into BIPAP (see below). These settings resulted in a mean airway pressure of 17 cm H_2O on APRV compared with 15 cm H_2O on IMV. These results suggest that the main benefit of APRV may be the reduction in peak airway pressure rather than mean airway pressure, a conclusion which confirms the similarity of APRV to inverse ratio ventilation.

113

Biphasic positive airway pressure ventilation (BIPAP). Another modification of CPAP is biphasic positive airway pressure ventilation. This permits the patient to breathe spontaneously at high and low positive pressures, which are alternated at slow respiratory frequencies (fig 5.2). The breathing system is similar to that used for APRV except that the solenoid valve is connected to a separate PEEP valve. The Dräger Evita ventilator may also be used to provide this mode. It is claimed that this technique provides good alveolar ventilation without sacrificing oxygenation.[28] An even more recently introduced technique is intermittent mandatory pressure release ventilation (IMPRV), in which airway pressure is released synchronously with the patient's expiration.[29] This requires a specially designed ventilator (the César).

Insufflation, apnoeic diffusion respiration, and continuous flow ventilation

In 1667 Hooke reported that life could be sustained in open chest dogs by blowing a constant stream of air into the lungs and allowing it to flow out through a series of puncture holes in the lung.[30] In 1909 Meltzer and Auer described similar experiments in which a continuous stream of air was delivered to the tracheal bifurcation by a tube and then allowed to escape through the tracheostomy incision.[31] In dogs with an open chest it was observed that the lungs were held distended and motionless but the dog survived. These observations led to the use of a narrow bore tracheal catheter for administering inhalational anaesthetic agents to patients, but under these circumstances shallow breathing continued unless anaesthesia was excessively deep. The insufflation technique was displaced by the use of the wide bore tracheal tube some 15 years after its introduction.

The phenomenon of apnoeic diffusion respiration was described in 1944[32] and subsequently investigated in humans.[33] The lungs are first washed out with oxygen and then connected to a reservoir of this gas. As oxygen is absorbed into the blood it generates a mass flow from the mouth to the alveoli so that arterial oxygenation is maintained during apnoea. The limitation is that CO_2 is not removed. Since apnoea results in an increase in arterial PCO_2 of 0.4–0.8 kPa/min (3–6 mm Hg/min) the technique can be used with safety for only 5–10 minutes in humans. Although the method was at one time used routinely for bronchoscopy and laryngoscopy under general anaesthesia, it is now used only for the short term treatment of airway emergencies.

The demonstration that high frequency oscillation (see below) provided adequate gas exchange with tidal volumes less than the dead space reawakened interest in the use of constant flow ventilation, and great interest was aroused when it was shown that normal blood gases could be maintained in apnoeic dogs by directing a continuous flow of oxygen into each bronchus.[34] High flow rates of gas were required, however, and although flows could be reduced by placing the tips of the catheters further down the bronchi, this carried a risk of overinflating localised areas of lung. Further studies of this technique in humans have shown that very high flow rates are required (1–1.5 l/kg body weight/min), and even these fail to prevent an increase in PCO_2.[35] The probable explanation for the failure of the technique in humans and some other species is that collateral ventilation is much less than in the dog. Recently it has been shown that dead space may be reduced by delivering a flow of fresh gas to the carina during mechanical ventilation; however, the dead space in the trachea is only a small proportion of the total dead space in patients with acute lung disease, so the benefits seem marginal.[36]

High frequency ventilation

Physiology

High frequency ventilation is usually defined as ventilation at frequencies of more than four times the normal frequency, but the range varies from 60 to 2400 bpm (1–40 Hz) depending on the technique used. The aim of high frequency ventilation is to reduce peak airway pressures by reducing tidal volume. If physiological dead space were to remain constant when tidal volume was reduced, ventilation would become progressively less efficient since the dead space would constitute a greater proportion of each breath. Minute volume would therefore have to be increased linearly to compensate for the increased proportion of wasted ventilation (fig 5.3). Finally, a point would be reached when the tidal volume equalled the dead space, so that alveolar ventilation would be zero. It is now known that this simple relation does not hold in clinical practice, and that dead space tends to decrease with tidal volume.

Studies of this problem have yielded variable results. Although species differences may account for some of this variability, most of it is due to methodological differences.[37] However, in one study of anaesthetised, intubated patients ventilated with a purpose built ventilator with low internal compliance, physiological dead space decreased as tidal volume was decreased when frequency was increased from 15 to 60 bpm, but from 80–120 bpm dead space was unchanged. Anatomical dead space (calculated from end tidal CO_2 measurements) changed in parallel with physiological dead space and reached a minimum of 1 ml/kg, and the ratio of dead space to tidal volume increased from 0.37 at 15 bpm to 0.73 at 120 bpm.[38] The decrease in dead space could be due to incomplete washout of the airways at the smaller tidal volumes,[39] but there is also evidence that it is due to augmented mixing of the inspired gas with the residual gas in the conducting airways. This probably results from the higher gas velocities associated with the increased minute volumes required at low tidal volumes.[40]

115

The above observations relate to the use of tidal volumes greater than the anatomical dead space. However, CO_2 elimination may still be adequate even when tidal volumes are less than the anatomical dead space, and at frequencies above 3 Hz additional mechanisms come into play. Proximally situated alveoli are probably ventilated directly, but most of the gas exchange seems to occur by augmented dispersion – that is, increased mixing of gases within the bronchial tree. Among the mechanisms causing this are convective streaming due to asymmetry of flow profiles induced by airway bifurcation; turbulent and laminar dispersion; and convective mixing in the conducting airways due to recirculation of gas among alveolar units with different time constants.[41] These create complex mixing patterns which enable the respiratory gases to pass rapidly from a region of high concentration to one of low. However, the process is relatively inefficient. Whereas CO_2 elimination at normal tidal volume is governed by the product of frequency and tidal volume, at very high frequencies it depends on the product of frequency and the square of tidal volume.[42]

Oxygenation during all forms of high frequency ventilation is directly related to mean alveolar pressure, which in turn governs lung volume.[43] Although mean alveolar pressure is closely related to mean airway pressure at low frequencies of ventilation, this relation no longer holds at high frequen-

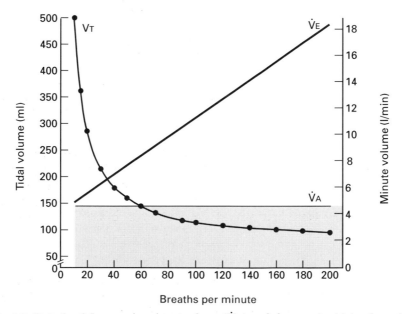

Fig 5.3 Calculated increase in minute volume ($\dot{V}E$) and decrease in tidal volume (VT) required to eliminate CO_2 output of 200 ml/min with increasing frequency. Dead space of 70 ml does not change with frequency; alveolar ventilation ($\dot{V}A$) required to maintain a normal PCO_2 is 4.3 l/min (shaded area).

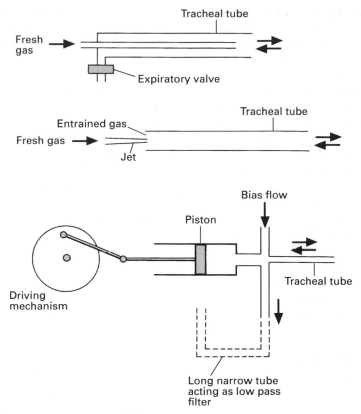

Fig 5.4 High frequency ventilation systems: (top) high frequency positive pressure ventilator; (centre) jet ventilator; (bottom) high frequency oscillator. Long, narrow tube acts as high impedance to oscillatory flow but allows CO_2 to be removed by bias flow.

cies because of the presence of gas trapping. This is why early comparisons of oxygenation at the same mean airway pressure showed better oxygenation with HFV than with conventional forms of ventilation. Since mean alveolar pressure is also directly related to mean intrathoracic pressure, cardiac output may be less than that predicted from mean airway pressure during HFV.

Techniques

The three basic techniques of high frequency ventilation are classified according to the method used to deliver the gas to the lungs (fig 5.4). In high frequency positive pressure ventilation (HFPPV) square wave pulses of gas are delivered into the trachea through a 0.5–1.0 cm internal diameter tube at frequencies of 60–120 bpm and there is little or no entrainment of other gases. Tidal volumes are in the range of 3–5 ml/kg and expiration is passive.

117

With high frequency jet ventilation (HFJV) the pulses are delivered at high velocities through a 1–2 mm diameter tube at frequencies of 1–5 Hz. The jet tube is usually incorporated into the wall of a special tracheal tube, but the inspired gas may also be delivered through a 14 or 16 gauge cannula (internal diameter 2.0 or 1.7 mm) which can be inserted through the cricothyroid membrane. The tidal volume is governed primarily by the jet flow rate, but this may be augmented by entrainment of ambient gas, which occurs mainly at the beginning of inspiration, or decreased by the spillage of gas ("blow back") which occurs towards the end of inspiration. Expiration is again passive.

In high frequency oscillation (HFO) the gas in the trachea is caused to mix with a bias flow of fresh gas by being oscillated to and fro at frequencies of 7–40 Hz. Both inspiration and expiration are active as they are governed by the oscillator. Tidal volumes are difficult to measure but are typically less than the volume of the airways. There are also a number of commercially available devices which superimpose high frequency oscillations on conventional mechanical ventilation wave forms, and an even more recent development is the application of high frequency oscillation to the outside of the chest during spontaneous breathing.

High frequency positive pressure ventilation was originally developed to reduce the respiratory fluctuations in blood pressure during animal experiments.[44] Later it became apparent that the reduced respiratory excursion could be of value during surgical procedures. The introduction of jet ventilation represented a major advance as it enabled controlled ventilation to be used in situations where it was not possible to make an airtight connection with the lung (laryngoscopy, bronchoscopy, and reconstruction of the trachea, for example). Again, the decreased tidal volume associated with the use of increased frequencies was seen as a potential advantage during surgical procedures, and it was also realised that the reduction in peak inflation pressures might be of value in minimising lung damage in adult or neonatal patients who required ventilatory support. The development of high frequency oscillation provided the ultimate in tidal volume reduction and has been shown to reduce lung damage in lung lavage models of the neonatal respiratory distress syndrome.[45] However, the clinical application of the technique has been limited.

High frequency positive pressure ventilation. HFPPV was the first technique to be developed. In the original technique, pulses of gas were delivered into an insufflation catheter placed within the tracheal tube. Expired gases passed out through a constant leak or a pneumatic valve system.[46] This arrangement reduced dead space and compressed gas volume to a minimum. It was found that at a frequency of 60 bpm peak pressures were about 65% of those generated at 20 bpm. Later studies in patients showed that there was a reduction in the effective dead space as tidal volume was reduced with increases in frequency to 60 or 80 bpm, but thereafter there was a linear increase in ventilation volume with frequency so that minute volumes of 20–30 l/min were required at 200 bpm.[47] With a fixed ratio of inspiratory to expiratory time, expiratory time is decreased as frequency is increased. This results in an increase in end expiratory lung volume, an increase in peak and mean intrathoracic pressures, and a reduction in cardiac output.[48] There is therefore little to be gained by ventilating at frequencies in excess of 60–80 bpm, even in patients with normal lungs. In patients with increased airway resistance gas trapping occurs at lower frequencies.

The technique has been used for bronchoscopy, laryngoscopy, and microlaryngeal surgery.[46] It has also been used for treating neonatal respiratory distress.[49]

High frequency jet ventilation. The use of jet ventilation at normal frequencies during bronchoscopy was pioneered by Sanders.[50] Transtracheal jet ventilation at frequencies from 20 to 200 bpm was first used in dogs by Klain and Smith[51] and HFJV was later used for laryngoscopy, the gas being delivered through a 3–4 mm internal diameter tube inserted through the larynx.[52] Supraglottic injection has proved to be of even more value, since it enables the pharynx to be kept free of combustible material during laser surgery.[53]

In a jet ventilator, square wave pulses of gas from a high pressure source are delivered to the jet tube at frequencies of 1–5 Hz, the upper limit of frequency being set by the response time of the solenoid, fluidic, or pneumatic valves that are used to control the flow, and the compressible volume within the delivery system. The ratio of inspiratory to expiratory time is usually adjustable from 1:1 to 1:5, and the tidal volume is set by varying the driving pressure, which is usually around 3–4 bar (45–60 psi) and, to a lesser extent, the duration of inspiration.

The jet of gas entrains ambient gas in the early part of inspiration, but as the pressure in the trachea increases, the flow of gas entering the lungs decreases and the excess gas (the "blowback" volume) escapes to the atmosphere. The jet thus functions as a constant pressure generator, flow into the lungs being maximal at the beginning of inspiration and then decreasing to zero. As a result an increase in inspiratory time does not produce a proportional increase in tidal volume. With such a pressure generator tidal volume depends on the compliance and airway resistance. However, since dead space does not decrease in proportion to tidal volume as frequency is increased, there must be a compensatory increase in minute volume. Furthermore, since the proportion of each minute available for inspiration is fixed, this must result in higher gas flow rates and higher pressure differences between the mouth and alveoli, so that a change in airway resistance has a proportionally greater effect on the volume of gas delivered than it does at normal frequencies.

119

The characteristics of the jet depend on the driving pressure, the internal diameter of the jet tube, and the geometry of the space into which the jet discharges.[54] For ventilation during laryngoscopy the jet tube usually consists of a stiff catheter with an internal diameter of 2–3 mm which is inserted through the vocal cords for a distance of 5–8 cm. For transtracheal ventilation a 14 or 16 gauge plastic catheter is used (internal diameter 2.0 or 1.7 mm). In both these situations it is vital that a free expiratory pathway is ensured at all times. Failure to do so can result in severe barotrauma.

For longer applications it is usual to use a special tracheal tube that incorporates both the jet tube and a separate tube for measuring tracheal pressure. This tube can be connected via a T piece to a high flow of humidified fresh gas so that the entrained gas has an appropriate oxygen concentration. The proportion of entrained gas is usually small (about 10–20% of the tidal volume), and further humidification is required. The most practical way of achieving this is by nebulising water into the jet flow.[55] PEEP can be applied by placing a threshold resistor on the outlet of the bias flow tube, but as the use of high frequencies results in the development of intrinsic PEEP there is seldom any indication for the addition of extrinsic PEEP.

The technique has three major disadvantages. Firstly, large minute volumes are required to compensate for the increased dead space to tidal volume ratio. Since the proportion of each minute that is devoted to inspiration is constant (normally 20–30%) this means that jet velocities may approach 60–80 l/min at 200 bpm. It is extremely difficult to humidify gas at such high flow rates, and if the jet impinges directly on the tracheal mucosa it can cause severe damage.[56] In the absence of adequate humidity, secretions become inspissated and cooling of the patient occurs.

The second disadvantage is that it is difficult to set and maintain the correct level of ventilation: the delivered volume can only be measured by using special techniques;[57] the jet functions as a pressure generator; and small alterations in the position of the jet within the airway may affect the amount of entrainment or blowback. Changes in the magnitude of entrainment also affect the inspired gas concentrations if the ambient gas composition differs from that delivered by the jet. As these variables are constantly changing, frequent estimations of PCO_2 are required. Few gas analysers have an adequate frequency response to provide accurate measurements of end tidal CO_2 at breathing frequencies above 60 bpm, but the end tidal plateau resulting from the third of several interposed deep breaths provides a good approximation to arterial PCO_2.[58]

The third disadvantage is the development of gas trapping at the higher frequencies. This can be detected only by measurement of mean airway pressure during regular interruption of the cycle, or by using an inductance plethysmograph to display the increase in lung volume.

HFJV has been used for long term ventilatory support in patients with severe acute lung disease, but a number of trials have failed to show any advantages over conventional methods.[59] It has also been used in an attempt to reduce the air leak in patients with a bronchopleural fistula, though there is little evidence that the use of HFJV decreases mortality.[60] HFJV is now usually reserved for specialist anaesthetic applications such as a difficult intubation and for operations on the larynx or trachea.[61]

High frequency oscillation (HFO). This technique was introduced by Lunkenheimer in 1972.[62] The oscillator usually consists of a sine wave pump or loudspeaker system which produces a stroke volume of 1–4 ml/kg at a frequency of 7–30 Hz. A steady flow of fresh, humidified gas crosses the oscillating gas stream so that the oscillating gas is continuously refreshed. The exhaled gas leaves through a long, narrow tube which provides a low resistance to the steady gas flow but a high impedance to the oscillatory flow, so acting as a crude low pass filter. It is difficult to know how much of the imparted oscillation is lost into this system, and under some circumstances resonance may cause the oscillations in the lung to exceed those in the oscillator.

CO_2 clearance is variable but roughly related to frequency and to the square of tidal volume, so that minute volumes at 15 Hz are about 10 times those required during conventional mechanical ventilation.[42, 63] As with HFJV, CO_2 clearance is reduced by an increase in airway resistance, since this reduces the proportion of the pump stroke volume that reaches the alveoli.

High frequency oscillation is a highly sophisticated technique which requires skilled supervision since small changes in airway resistance or ventilator setting can produce large variations in lung volume and gas exchange. High frequency oscillation has been used with success in treating neonatal respiratory distress, and there is some evidence that, after recruitment of previously closed alveoli, alveolar expansion may be maintained at a lower mean airway pressure than with conventional ventilation. However, mean intra-alveolar pressure may well exceed mean airway pressure because of differences in inspiratory and expiratory airway resistances and the short expiratory period, and care must be taken to ensure that overinflation does not occur. The technique has been reported to improve blood gases in newborn infants with persistent pulmonary hypertension, pneumonia, meconium aspiration, the respiratory distress syndrome, or diaphragmatic hernia.[63]

Despite the theoretical advantages, a recent controlled trial of its use in respiratory failure in preterm infants failed to show any difference in mortality or complications between those treated with HFO and those treated with a conventional IMV technique.[64] However, very few of the centres had previous experience of HFO and the trial has been criticised by two of the main proponents of the technique. They claim that the success of the technique depends on the recruitment of collapsed areas of lung by the use of high mean airway pressure in the early stages of treatment, pressures then being reduced as the lung condition improves.[65] It is postulated that the high mean airway pressures used in the early stages of treatment with HFO prevent the repeated opening and closing of alveoli which, it is believed, lead to further lung damage, and also that the high alveolar pressures are not transmitted through the stiff lung to the pleural space, so that there is little reduction in cardiac output.[66]

The high mean pressure/lung volume technique is being subjected to a further randomised clinical trial, but preliminary studies suggest that this technique provides a useful alternative to extracorporeal membrane oxygenation in infants who do not respond to conventional treatment for the respiratory distress syndrome;[66] that it decreases the incidence of chronic respiratory disease observed after recovery;[67] and that it may be of use in other types of severe lung disease encountered in paediatric patients.[68] However, improvements in other treatments such as surfactant replacement therapy[69] may well reduce the indications for this form of treatment.

High frequency chest wall oscillation. Experiments have shown that normal gas exchange can be secured in apnoeic animals by placing the whole body within a chamber and then vibrating the air within it.[70] In humans, chest wall vibration has been used to assist CO_2 clearance in spontaneously breathing subjects by applying rapid oscillations to a cuff surrounding the thorax,[71] but the pressure exerted by the cuff causes a reduction in functional residual capacity.[72] This problem can be overcome by surrounding the chest with a cuirass and applying a constant subatmospheric pressure with superimposed oscillations to the air contained within. By further reducing the absolute pressure in the chamber, it is possible to produce increases in lung volume comparable to those produced by CPAP. A commercial version of such a device (the Hayek oscillator) has been shown to assist CO_2 removal in patients with chronic obstructive airways disease.[73]

Mixed CMV-HFV. Various forms of high frequency ventilation have been superimposed on conventional mechanical ventilation and several reports have claimed that the combination improves gas exchange. In one randomised trial in patients with ARDS, those treated with a high frequency percussive system (which superimposed flow oscillations on both inspiration and expiration) reached the therapeutic end point at a lower level of CPAP and mean airway pressure than those treated with IMV. However, there were no differences in mortality, duration of stay in the intensive care unit or hospital, or any other variable, between the two groups.[74]

Extracorporeal gas exchange

Extracorporeal membrane oxygenation

The obvious method of resting the lung is to take over gas exchange with an artificial lung. Early attempts used extracorporeal membrane oxygenation (ECMO) with a membrane lung, thereby maintaining both O_2 and CO_2 exchange by artificial means. This was technically difficult and expensive in terms of equipment and staffing, and when compared with conventional CMV with PEEP in a carefully designed randomised trial ECMO was shown to have no effect on mortality.[75] However, it has been used widely in the treatment of neonates with meconium aspiration, the neonatal respiratory distress syndrome, and persistent pulmonary hypertension[76] and shown to increase survival rates to approximately 85%, though the treatment of babies with persistent air leaks, diaphragmatic hernia, or sepsis has not been so successful.[77, 78] A small but finite incidence of neurological damage is associated with the cannulation of the carotid artery and internal jugular vein,[79] but the technique is of great value in situations where the period of respiratory support is unlikely to be unduly prolonged. As would be expected with such severe disease, there is a high incidence of chronic lung disease in those submitted to this form of treatment.[80] ECMO has also been used in paediatric patients with moderate success.[81]

Extracorporeal CO_2 removal $(ECCO_2R)$

In 1978 Gattinoni and colleagues introduced the revolutionary new technique of extracorporeal CO_2 removal.[82] In this technique the two aspects of gas exchange are separated, oxygenation being achieved by the lung and CO_2 exchange by a veno-venous extracorporeal circuit with a membrane lung optimised for CO_2 removal. The advantage of this arrangement is that, theoretically, all the CO_2 production can be removed with a blood flow of 1–2 l/min, whereas with ECMO the whole of the cardiac output has to perfuse the membrane lung. The reduced extracorporeal flow reduces blood damage and enables percutaneous catheters to be used; the recent introduction of heparinised circuits[83] has facilitated control of anticoagulation and greatly reduced bleeding, which was one of the major problems with ECMO. Since CO_2 elimination is no longer a problem the lung can be maintained under optimal conditions for repair. It is not known what these are, but current practice is to use low frequency (4–6 bpm) pressure controlled ventilation (25–35 cm H_2O) and a PEEP of 7–15 cm H_2O, inspired oxygen being reduced below 50% when arterial PO_2 exceeds 8 kPa (60 mm Hg).

The membrane lungs used in clinical practice are not optimised for CO_2 removal, so that blood flows of 2–4 l/min often have to be used. With these flows there is a significant increase in mixed venous PO_2 which helps to counteract the impaired oxygen uptake in the lungs resulting from the high levels of intrapulmonary shunt in patients with ARDS. Centres specialising in this technique claim a survival rate of 50–60% in very severe cases of the syndrome. However, a recent randomised, controlled trial in patients who fulfilled the entry criteria for the ECMO trial[75] failed to show any improvement in survival compared with those treated with pressure controlled inverse ratio ventilation.[84]

Intravascular gas exchange

The most recent advance is an intravascular gas exchange device. This is, in effect, a hollow fibre membrane lung contained within a catheter that can be passed into the inferior vena cava. The fibres are flushed with oxygen so that oxygen and carbon dioxide can be exchanged with the venous blood. The catheter has an anticoagulant coating and it is anticipated that it can remain in situ for days. Current models seem to be capable of providing 10–25% of the body's gas exchange requirements, but there are some complications.[85] The device may also create an obstruction to venous return, and one recent report suggested that any benefits in terms of gas exchange were offset by a decrease in cardiac index and oxygen transport.[86]

Conclusions

High frequency ventilation was a promising development, and provided a great deal of physiological interest, but it proved disappointing in clinical practice. The basic problem with HFPPV and HFJV is that, although there is some reduction in dead space with tidal volume, there is an approximately linear increase in required minute volume with increasing frequency. Humidification is difficult, and the correct ventilator setting can be determined only by examining the end tidal CO_2 during interposed deep breaths or by repeated blood gas analysis. Jet ventilation has the additional disadvantage that the jet functions as a pressure generator. High flow rates are required to produce the large minute volumes required at the higher frequencies so that there is a large pressure drop down the airways, and entrainment and blow back are considerably influenced by small changes in airway resistance. Gas trapping occurs at frequencies above 1 Hz and increases the mean intra-alveolar pressure and lung volume. This improves oxygenation but it also decreases cardiac output. Careful monitoring of mean airway pressure or end expiratory lung volume is therefore required. Although jet ventilation at normal or slightly increased frequencies is useful for special problems in anaesthetic practice, current evidence does not support long term use of either HFJV or HFO.

Great progress has been made in simplifying the techniques of extracorporeal support during the past 20 years, and many of the earlier problems such as bleeding, anticoagulation, and blood damage have been largely overcome by

124

the use of percutaneous cannulations, heparin bonded surfaces, and centrifugal pumps. However, repair in a lung severely damaged by ARDS may take many weeks, and maintenance of support for this period throws a heavy load on scarce resources. There seems to be no doubt that ECMO is very successful in selected neonates with severe respiratory distress, but there is still no incontrovertible evidence that extracorporeal CO_2 removal in adults with ARDS significantly reduces mortality.

1 Leroy J. Recherches sur l'asphyxie. *J Physiol exper Pathol* 1827;7:45–65 and 1828;8:97–135.
2 Macklin CC. Transport of air along sheaths of pulmonic blood vessels from alveoli to mediastinum. Clinical implications. *Arch Intern Med* 1939;64:913–26.
3 Northway WH, Rosan RC, Porter DY. Pulmonary disease following respiratory therapy of hyaline membrane disease. *N Engl J Med* 1967;276:357–68.
4 Nash G, Blennerhassett JB, Pontoppidan H. Pulmonary lesions associated with oxygen therapy and artificial ventilation. *N Engl J Med* 1967;276:368–74.
5 Johnson TH, Altman AR. Pulmonary interstitial gas: first sign of barotrauma due to PEEP therapy. *Crit Care Med* 1979;7:532 5.
6 Kumar A, Pontoppidan H, Falke KJ, Wilson RS, Laver MB. Pulmonary barotrauma during mechanical ventilation. *Crit Care Med* 1973;1:181–6.
7 Albelda SM, Gefter WB, Kelley MA, Epstein DM, Miller WT. Ventilator-induced subpleural air cysts: clinical, radiographic, and pathologic significance. *Am Rev Respir Dis* 1983;127:360–5.
8 Slavin G, Nunn JF, Crow J, Doré CJ. Bronchiolectasis – a complication of artificial ventilation. *BMJ* 1982;285:931–4.
9 Baeza OR, Wagner RB, Lowery BD. Pulmonary hyperinflation. A form of barotrauma during mechanical ventilation. *J Thorac Cardiovasc Surg* 1975;70:790–803.
10 Kolobow T, Moretti MP, Fumagalli R, Mascheroni D, Prato P, Chen V, *et al*. Severe impairment in lung function induced by high peak airway pressure during mechanical ventilation. *Am Rev Repir Dis* 1987;135:312–5.
11 Parker JC, Hernandez LA, Peevy KJ. Mechanisms of ventilator-induced lung injury. *Crit Care Med* 1993;21:131–43.
12 Dreyfuss D, Saumon G. Barotrauma is volutrauma, but which volume is the one responsible? *Intensive Care Med* 1992;18:139–41.
13 Gattinoni L, Pesenti A. ARDS: the non-homogeneous lung; facts and hypothesis. *Intensive Crit Care Digest* 1987;6:1–4.
14 Gattinoni L, Pesenti A, Bombino M, Baglioni S, Rivolta M, Rossi F, *et al*. Relationships between lung computed tomographic density, gas exchange, and PEEP in acute respiratory failure. *Anesthesiology* 1988;69:824–32.
15 Hickling KG, Henderson SJ, Jackson R. Low mortality associated with low volume pressure limited ventilation with permissive hypercapnia in severe adult respiratory distress syndrome. *Intensive Care Med* 1990;16:372–7.
16 Hickling KG, Howard R. A retrospective survey of treatment and mortality in aspiration pneumonia. *Intensive Care Med* 1988;14:617–22.
17 Pesenti A. Target blood gases during ARDS ventilatory management. *Intensive Care Med* 1990;16:349–51.
18 Watson WE. Observations on physiological dead space during intermittent positive pressure respiration. *Br J Anaesth* 1962;34:502–8.
19 Reynolds EOR. Effect of alterations in mechanical ventilator settings on pulmonary gas exchange in hyaline membrane disease. *Arch Dis Child* 1971;46:152–9.
20 Herman S, Reynolds EOR. Methods for improving oxygenation in infants mechanically ventilated for severe hyaline membrane disease. *Arch Dis Child* 1973;48:612–7.
21 Boros SJ. Variations in inspiratory:expiratory ratio and airway pressure wave form during mechanical ventilation: the significance of mean airway pressure. *J Pediatr* 1979;94:114–7.
22 Marcy TW, Marini JJ. Inverse ratio ventilation in ARDS. Rationale and implementation. *Chest* 1991;100:494–504.

125

23 Cole AGH, Weller SF, Sykes MK. Inverse ratio ventilation compared with PEEP in adult respiratory failure. *Intensive Care Med* 1984;**10**:227–32.
24 Tharratt RS, Allen RP, Albertson TE. Pressure controlled inverse ratio ventilation in severe adult respiratory failure. *Chest* 1988;**94**:755–62.
25 Duncan SR, Rizk NW, Raffin TA. Inverse ratio ventilation. PEEP in disguise? *Chest* 1987;**92**:390–1.
26 Stock MC, Downs JB, Frolicher DA. Airway pressure release ventilation. *Crit Care Med* 1987;**15**:462–6.
27 Räsänen J, Cane RD, Downs JB, Hurst JM, Jousela IT, Kirby RR, et al. Airway pressure release ventilation during acute lung injury: a prospective multicenter trial. *Crit Care Med* 1991;**19**:1234–41.
28 Hörmann Ch, Baum M, Putensen Ch, Mutz NJ, Benzer H. Biphasic positive airway pressure (BIPAP) – a new mode of ventilatory support. *Eur J Anaesthesiol* 1994;**11**:37–42.
29 Rouby J-J, Ben Ameur M, Jawish A, Cherif A, Andreev A, Dreux S, et al. Continuous positive airway pressure (CPAP) vs intermittent mandatory pressure release ventilation (IMPRV) in patients with acute respiratory failure. *Intensive Care Med* 1992;**18**:69–75.
30 Hook R. An account of an experiment made by Mr Hook, of preserving animals alive by blowing through their lungs with bellows. *Phil Trans Roy Soc* 1667;**2**:539–40.
31 Meltzer SJ, Auer J. Continuous respiration without respiratory movements. *J Exp Med* 1909;**11**:622–5.
32 Draper WB, Whitehead RW. Diffusion respiration in the dog anesthetized by pentothal sodium. *Anesthesiology* 1944;**5**:262–73.
33 Holmdahl MH. Pulmonary uptake of oxygen, acid base metabolism, and circulation during prolonged apnoea. *Acta Chir Scand* 1956;**212**:1–128.
34 Lehnert BE, Oberdörster G, Slutsky AS. Constant-flow ventilation of apneic dogs. *J Appl Physiol* 1982;**53**:483–9.
35 Breen PH, Sznajder JI, Morrison P, Hatch D, Wood LDH, Craig DB. Constant flow ventilation in anesthetized patients: efficacy and safety. *Anesth Analg* 1986;**65**:1161–9.
36 Ravenscraft SA, Burke WC, Nahum A, Adams AB, Nakos G, Marcy TW, et al. Tracheal gas insufflation augments CO_2 clearance during mechanical ventilation. *Am Rev Respir Dis* 1993;**148**:345–51.
37 Weinmann GG, Mitzner W, Permutt S. Physiological dead space during high-frequency ventilation in dogs. *J Appl Physiol* 1984;**57**:881–7.
38 Chakrabarti MK, Gordon G, Whitwam JG. Relationship between tidal volume and deadspace during high frequency ventilation. *Br J Anaesth* 1986;**58**:11–7.
39 Briscoe WA, Forster RE, Comroe JH. Alveolar ventilation at very low tidal volumes. *J Appl Physiol* 1954;**7**:27–30.
40 Eriksson I. The role of conducting airways in gas exchange during high-frequency ventilation – a clinical and theoretical analysis. *Anesth Analg* 1982;**61**:483–9.
41 Chang HK, Mechanisms of gas transport during ventilation by high frequency oscillation. *J Appl Physiol* 1984;**56**:553–63.
42 Kolton M. A review of high frequency oscillation. *Can Anaesth Soc J* 1984;**31**:416–29.
43 Rouby JJ, Fusciardi J, Bourgain JL, Viars P. High-frequency jet ventilation in postoperative respiratory failure: determinants of oxygenation. *Anesthesiology* 1983;**59**:281–7.
44 Jonzon A, Öberg PA, Sedin G, Sjöstrand U. High frequency positive-pressure ventilation by endotracheal insufflation. *Acta Anaesthesiol Scand* 1971;**43**(suppl):1–43.
45 Sykes MK. Does mechanical ventilation damage the lung? *Acta Anaesthesiol Scand* 1991;**35**(suppl 95):35–9.
46 Sjöstrand U, ed. Experimental and clinical evaluation of high-frequency positive-pressure ventilation. *Acta Anaesthesiol Scand* 1977;**64**(suppl):1–178.
47 Borg U, Eriksson I, Sjöstrand U. High frequency positive pressure ventilation (HFPPV): a review based on its use during bronchoscopy and for laryngoscopy and microlaryngeal surgery under general anesthesia. *Anesth Analg* 1980;**59**:594–603.
48 Chakrabarti MK, Sykes MK. Cardiorespiratory effects of high frequency intermittent positive pressure ventilation in the dog. *Br J Anaesth* 1980;**52**:475–81.
49 Bland RD, Kim MH, Light MS, Woodson JL. High frequency mechanical ventilation in severe hyaline membrane disease – an alternative treatment? *Crit Care Med* 1980;**8**:275–80.
50 Sanders RD. Two ventilating attachments for bronchoscopes. *Del Med J* 1967;**39**:170–5.

51 Klain M, Smith RB. High frequency percutaneous transtracheal jet ventilation. *Crit Care Med* 1977;**5**:280–7.
52 Babinski M, Smith RB, Klain M. High frequency jet ventilation for laryngoscopy. *Anesthesiology* 1980;**52**:178–80.
53 Hermens JM, Bennett MJ, Hirshman CA. Anesthesia for laser surgery. *Anesth Analg* 1983;**62**:218–29.
54 Young JD, Dorrington KL. Peak airway pressure during high frequency jet ventilation: theory and measurement. *Br J Anaesth* 1988;**61**:601–5.
55 Smith BE. The Penlon Bromsgrove high frequency jet ventilator for adult and paediatric use. A solution to the problems of humidification. *Anaesthesia* 1985;**40**:790–6.
56 Boros SJ, Mammel MC, Lewallen PK, Coleman JM, Gordon MJ, Ophoven J. Necrotizing tracheobronchitis: a complication of high frequency ventilation. *J Pediatr* 1986;**109**:95–100.
57 Young DJ, Sykes MK. A method for measuring tidal volume during high frequency jet ventilation. *Br J Anaesth* 1988;**61**:601–5.
58 Mortimer AJ, Cannon DP, Sykes MK. Estimation of arterial PCO_2 during high frequency jet ventilation. *Br J Anaesth* 1987;**59**:240–6.
59 Standiford TJ, Morganroth ML. High frequency ventilation. *Chest* 1989;**96**:1380–9.
60 Bishop MJ, Benson MS, Sato P, Pierson DJ. Comparison of high frequency jet ventilation with conventional mechanical ventilation for bronchopleural fistula. *Anesth Analg* 1987;**66**:833–8.
61 Giunta F, Chiaranda M, Manani G, Giron CP. Clinical uses of high frequency jet ventilation in anaesthesia. *Br J Anaesth* 1989;**63**:102–6S.
62 Lunkenheimer PP, Rafflenbeul W, Keller H, Frank I, Dickhut HH, Fuhrmann C. Application of transtracheal pressure oscillations as a modification of "diffusion respiration". *Br J Anaesth* 1972;**44**:627.
63 Froese AB, Bryan AC. High frequency ventilation. *Am Rev Respir Dis* 1987;**135**:1363–74.
64 HiFi study group. High-frequency oscillatory ventilation compared with conventional mechanical ventilation in the treatment of respiratory failure in preterm infants. *N Engl J Med* 1989;**320**:88–93.
65 Bryan AC, Froese AB. Reflections on the HiFi trial. *Pediatrics* 1991;**87**:565–7.
66 Arnold JH, Truog RD, Thompson JE, Fackler JC. High frequency oscillatory ventilation in pediatric respiratory failure. *Crit Care Med* 1993;**21**:272–8.
67 Clark RH, Gerstmann DR, Null DM, deLemos RA. Prospective randomized comparison of high-frequency oscillatory and conventional ventilation in respiratory distress syndrome. *Pediatrics* 1992;**89**:5–12.
68 Carter JM, Gerstmann DR, Clark RH, Snyder G, Cornish JD, Null DM, *et al.* High-frequency oscillatory ventilation and extracorporeal membrane oxygenation for the treatment of acute neonatal respiratory failure. *Pediatrics* 1990;**85**:159–64.
69 Speer CP, Robertson B, Curstedt T, Halliday HL, Compagnone D, Gefeller O, *et al.* Randomized European multicenter trial of surfactant replacement therapy for severe neonatal respiratory distress syndrome: single versus multiple doses of Curosurf. *Pediatrics* 1992;**89**:13–20.
70 Zidulka A, Gross D, Minami H, Vartian V, Chang HK. Ventilation by high-frequency chest wall compression in dogs with normal lungs. *Am Rev Respir Dis* 1983;**127**:709–13.
71 George RJD, Winter R, Flockton SJ, Geddes DM. Ventilatory saving by external chest wall compression or oral high-frequency oscillation in normal subjects and those with chronic airflow obstruction. *Clin Sci* 1985;**69**:349–59.
72 Calverley PMA, Chang HK, Vartian V, Zidulka A. High-frequency chest wall oscillation: assistance to ventilation in spontaneously breathing subjects. *Chest* 1986;**89**:218–23.
73 Spitzer SA, Fink G, Mittelman M. External high-frequency ventilation in severe chronic obstructive pulmonary disease. *Chest* 1993;**104**:1698–701.
74 Hurst JM, Branson RD, Davis K, Barrette RR, Adams KS. Comparison of conventional mechanical ventilation and high-frequency ventilation. A prospective, randomized trial in patients with respiratory failure. *Ann Surg* 1990;**211**:486–91.
75 Zapol WM, Snider MT, Hill JD, Fallat RJ, Bartlett RH, Edmunds LJ, *et al.* Extracorporeal membrane oxygenation in severe acute respiratory failure. A randomized prospective study. *JAMA* 1979;**242**:2193–6.
76 O'Rourke PP, Crone RK, Vacanti JP, Ware JH, Lillehei CW, Parad B, *et al.* Extracorporeal

127

membrane oxygenation and conventional medical therapy in neonates with persistent pulmonary hypertension of the newborn: a prospective randomized study. *Pediatrics* 1989;**84**:957–63.

77 Pearson GA, Firmin RK, Sosnowski A. Review. Neonatal extracorporeal oxygenation. *Br J Hosp Med* 1992;**47**:646–53.

78 Toomasian JM, Snedecor SM, Cornell RG, Cilley RE, Bartlett RH. National experience with extracorporeal membrane oxygenation for respiratory failure: data from 715 cases. *ASAIO Trans* 1988;**34**:130–47.

79 Campbell LA, Bunyapen C, Holmes GL, Howell CG, Kanto JP. Right common carotid artery ligation in extracorporeal membrane oxygenation. *J Pediatr* 1988;**113**:110–3.

80 Schwendeman CA, Clark RH, Yoder BA, Null DM, Gerstmann DR, et al. Frequency of chronic lung disease in infants with severe respiratory failure treated with high-frequency ventilation and/or extracorporeal membrane oxygenation. *Crit Care Med* 1992;**20**:372–7.

81 Moler FW, Custer JR, Bartlett RH, Palmisano J, Meliones JN, Delius RE, et al. Extracorporeal life support for pediatric respiratory failure. *Crit Care Med* 1992;**20**:1112–8.

82 Gattinoni L, Kolobow T, Tomlinson T, Iapichino G, Samaja M, White D, et al. Low-frequency positive pressure ventilation with extracorporeal CO_2 removal (LFPPV-ECCO$_2$R): an experimental study. *Anesth Analg* 1978;**57**:470–7.

83 Bindslev L, Böhm C, Jolin K, Jonzon KH, Olsson P, Ryniak S. Extracorporeal carbon dioxide removal performed with surface-heparinized equipment in patient with ARDS. *Acta Anaesthesiol Scand* 1991;**35**(Suppl 95):125–31.

84 Morris AH, Wallace CJ, Menlove RL, Clemmer TP, Orme JF, Weaver LK, et al. Randomized clinical trial of pressure-controlled inverse ratio ventilation and extracorporeal CO_2 removal for adult respiratory distress syndrome. *Am J Respir Crit Care Med* 1994;**149**:295–305.

85 High KM, Snider MY, Richard R, Russell GB, Stene JK, Campbell DB, et al. Clinical trials of an intravenous oxygenator in patients with adult respiratory distress syndrome. *Anesthesiology* 1992;**77**:856–63.

86 Gentilello LM, Jurkovich GJ, Gubler KD, Anardi DM, Heiskell R. The intravascular oxygenator (IVOX): preliminary results of a new means of performing extrapulmonary gas exchange. *J Trauma* 1993;**35**:399–404.

6 Modern ventilator technology

In the space available it is obviously impossible to provide a detailed description of every ventilator in common use. One well known ventilator will therefore be described in some detail and compared with four others in order to illustrate the functional differences. Table 6.1 summarises the flow waveforms which each machine is capable of generating, and Table 6.2 lists the four primary controls that have to be set on each ventilator to define the characteristics of the mandatory breath. The magnitude of the fifth variable, which may be peak flow rate, inspiratory to expiratory ratio, or inspiratory pause time, will depend on the chosen pattern of flow. A more detailed description of these and other ventilators is given in other publications[1-7] and the manufacturers' literature.

Siemens-Elema Servo 900 series

The Siemens-Elema Servoventilator was first described in 1972.[8] It was one of the first electronically controlled ventilators to be marketed and represented a breakthrough in ventilator design as it used the concept of servocontrol to produce the desired flow patterns.

The fundamental characteristic of any servocontrol system is that the measured output from the system is continuously compared with the preset value. If the output differs from the preset value the control signal is modified to return the output to the desired value. In the Servoventilator the output from a pressurised source of gas is controlled by an inspiratory valve

Table 6.1 *Electronic ventilators: availability of inspiratory flow waveforms in flow generation mode. All ventilators produce a decreasing flow pattern in the pressure generation mode*

Ventilator	Flow waveforms available			
	Constant	Sinusoidal	Increasing	Decreasing
Siemens-Elema 900C	+		+	
Hamilton Veolar	+	+	+	+
Engström Erica/Elvira	+		+	+
Puritan Bennett 7200	+	+		+
Dräger Evita	+			

Table 6.2 Variables affected by changing flow waveform during controlled ventilation with the flow generation mode

Ventilator	Controls				Variable
Siemens-Elema 900C	$\dot{V}_E$	f	$T_I\%$	$T_p\%$	$\dot{V}_I$
Hamilton Veolar	V_T	f	$T_I\%$	$T_p\%$	$\dot{V}_I$
Engström Erica	V_T	f	$T_I{:}T_E$	$\dot{V}_I$	T_p
Engström Elvira	V_T	f	T_p	$\dot{V}_I$	$T_I{:}T_E$
Dräger Evita	V_T	f	$T_I{:}T_E$	$\dot{V}_I$	T_p
Puritan Bennett 7200	V_T	f	T_p	$\dot{V}_I$	$T_I{:}T_E$

$\dot{V}_E$ = minute volume; V_T = tidal volume; f = respiratory rate; T_I = inspiratory time, T_E = expiratory time, and T_p = pause time (all expressed as % of respiratory cycle); $\dot{V}_I$ = inspiratory flow rate.

and a flow meter which measures the flow through it. The operator selects the tidal volume, the inspiratory time, and the inspiratory flow pattern and the logic unit then determines the pattern of gas flow that is required to satisfy these conditions.

At the onset of inspiration the inspiratory valve opens rapidly until the flow meter shows that this flow has been achieved. The flow is continuously measured by the flow meter and this measurement is then continuously compared with the desired pattern of flow. Any deviation between the set pattern of flow and the actual output from the valve activates the servomechanism, which then adjusts the valve opening to maintain the preset pattern of flow. Such a system is very flexible because it can produce a variety of flow patterns. It has the additional advantage that it may also be controlled by the pressure in the patient breathing system and thus may be used to generate CPAP and other spontaneous breathing modes. Variants of this system are now used in most of the modern ventilators.

The Servo 900C will be described since it is in widespread use and illustrates many of the principles found in the present generation of ventilators. It can be used with adults or children in the intensive therapy unit or in anaesthesia. The ventilator consists of two compartments, the lower containing an electronic unit, which carries out all the logic functions, and the upper an easily accessible pneumatic unit, which controls the gas flow to and from the patient. The pneumatic unit has three components: a gas reservoir and inspiratory and expiratory valve units (fig 6.1). The gas reservoir consists of a large, spring loaded bellows which maintains a constant driving pressure. This can be adjusted between 10 and 120 cm H_2O but is usually set 10–20 cm H_2O above the peak airway pressure. The reservoir pressure is displayed on an aneroid gauge on the front of the pneumatic unit.

There are two inputs to the bellows. One is a low pressure input, which is used when gases are being metered by wall flow meters or an anaesthetic machine, and the other is a high pressure inlet, which is usually attached to a high pressure oxygen-air blender. Gas flow from the high pressure inlet is

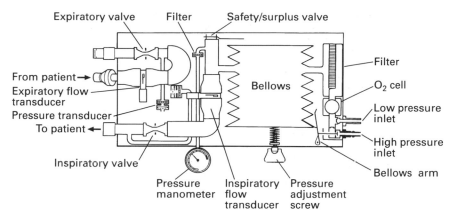

Fig 6.1   Siemens Servo 900C pneumatic system.

controlled by a valve that is designed to maintain a constant pressure and volume of gas in the bellows. There is also a combined safety/surplus valve which opens when the bellows becomes overfilled at low pressure or when the pressure exceeds 120 cm H_2O.

The gas from both inlets passes through an oxygen analyser and bacterial filter and leaves the bellows through the inspiratory flow meter and valve. The flow meter senses the difference in pressure across a linear resistance element. The valve consists of a silicone rubber tube which is compressed by two metal rods; one is fixed and the other can be moved in a series of steps by a stepper motor, each step corresponding to a change in flow of about 10%.

The logic unit calculates the instantaneous flow rate required to generate the tidal volume with the preset inspiratory time and flow pattern, and this is continually compared with the actual flow through the inspiratory valve. The valve orifice is then servocontrolled to reproduce the preset flow pattern. This system permits a reasonable control of the inspiratory flow pattern when the driving pressure is 10–20 cm H_2O higher than the peak airway pressure, but the flow pattern will not be maintained if the driving pressure is set too low or if a high airway pressure is required to inflate the lungs.

The gases returning from the patient pass through a similar valve and flow meter, but the flow meter is heated to about 60°C to prevent condensation on the resistance element. The pressures in both the inspiratory and expiratory tubes are measured by transducers, which are separated from the breathing system by bacterial filters. Both of the mechanical valves automatically open if a power failure occurs, thus allowing the patient to breathe spontaneously through the machine. Under these circumstances, rebreathing is prevented by a non-return valve situated at the outlet from the machine, but the patient will be exposed to a continuous positive pressure of approximately 15 cm H_2O.

131

Controls

Flow generator mode. The tidal volume is determined by the controls which set respiratory frequency (5–120 breaths/min) and minute volume (0.5–40 l/min) (fig 6.2). It is then necessary to set the "inspiratory time %" (the period during which gas is being driven into the patient, variable between 20% and 80% of the cycle) and the "inspiratory pause time %" (variable between 0% and 30%). The sum of these two is the inspiratory phase time, expressed as a percentage of the total cycle time. Thus with a frequency of 10 breaths/min (cycle time 6 seconds), an inspiratory time of 30%, and a pause time of 20% the inspiratory phase would last for 50% of the cycle (3 seconds). The inspiratory:expiratory ratio would thus be 1:1. As a safety feature the ventilator does not permit settings that would result in an inspiratory:expiratory ratio of more than 4:1. If, for example, the inspiratory time % were set to 70% and the pause time to 20%, the machine would cycle to expiration when the total inspiratory phase time exceeded 80%, thus shortening the pause time to 10%.

Three other controls require adjustment. The first is the "upper pressure limit." This is adjustable between 16 and 120 cm H_2O and would normally be set at around 60 cm H_2O when the machine is being used as a flow generator. If this limit is exceeded the ventilator behaves as a pressure cycled machine and cycles to expiration. The second is the control that gives a choice of constant or increasing flow during inspiration. This is active only when the machine is functioning as a flow generator, since the flow will always decrease exponentially when the machine is being used as a constant pressure generator. The third is the PEEP control. This provides an adjustable level between 0 and 50 cm H_2O, but there is a safety catch at 20 cm H_2O. The PEEP level is controlled by the expiratory valve, which closes progressively as the airway pressure falls towards the set level.

Pressure generator mode. Although a constant airway pressure could be generated by decreasing the pressure in the bellows to the desired level, the inspiratory valve system is normally used to maintain a fixed pressure level in the inspiratory circuit. The desired pressure level is set with the "inspiratory pressure level above PEEP" control, which allows for the need for a higher driving pressure when PEEP is used. Thus when PEEP is set at 5 cm H_2O and the inspiratory pressure level at 20 cm H_2O the ventilator will generate an airway pressure of 25 cm H_2O.

Other modes. The main control knob for ventilatory modes enables the machine to be set to deliver "volume controlled" breaths (flow generator mode), "volume control plus sigh" (a breath of twice the set tidal volume at intervals of 100 breaths), and "pressure control." The ventilator can also be programmed to produce a number of spontaneous breathing modes: "CPAP," "pressure support," and "SIMV," either alone or with pressure

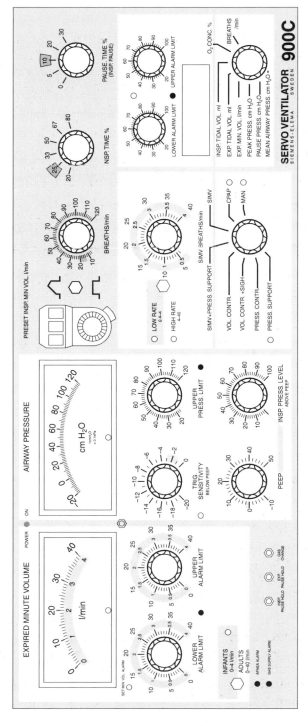

Fig. 6.2 *Control panel of Siemens Servo 900C (by courtesy Siemens plc Medical Engineering, Siemens House, Oldbury, Bracknell, Berkshire RG12 8FZ). The three special function buttons are situated under a flap at bottom left.*

support. The inspiratory phase is triggered by the patient induced reduction in pressure in the inspiratory tubing, and trigger sensitivity is set by the "trigger sensitivity below PEEP" control. This is adjustable between 0 and -20 cm H_2O.

When the main control is set to CPAP the patient can breath spontaneously through the system at the set PEEP level, the inspiratory and expiratory valves matching the gas flow to the patient's demands and controlling the direction of flow. When the "pressure support" mode is engaged the ventilator provides a constant pressure throughout inspiration, the level of pressure being controlled by the inspiratory pressure above PEEP control. The level of support may vary from a few cm H_2O (sufficient to overcome the resistance of tubes and humidifier) to a level of support high enough to produce a full tidal volume.

The flow pattern resulting from the use of this modality is governed by the patient, since the constant applied pressure is designed only to augment the patient's inspiratory efforts. Flow is terminated when the flow rate drops to 25% of the peak flow. However, if there is some other failure, such as a leak from the system, inspiration may be terminated when the airway pressure exceeds 3 cm H_2O above the PEEP level or when the inspiratory time exceeds 80% of the cycle time.

In the SIMV mode the patient breathes spontaneously but receives intermittent mandatory breaths with the characteristics defined by the other controls on the ventilator. The frequency of the mandatory breaths is then set with the "SIMV breaths/min" control. When the "SIMV + press support" mode is engaged the spontaneous breaths are subject to the degree of pressure support set on the "insp. press. level above PEEP" control.

Three special function buttons are located under a small flap. Two of these permit the operator to create a pause at the end of inspiration or expiration so that equilibrium measurements of airway pressure can be obtained for measurement of static compliance or intrinsic PEEP, and the third enables the system to be flushed after a change in inspired gas mixture.

Monitors and alarms

Analogue meters display airway pressure and expired volume, and there are controls to set the upper and lower alarm limits for volume. There are alarms for gas supply failure, oxygen concentration, and apnoea. A single digital display can be used for oxygen concentration; peak, pause or mean airway pressure; inspired or expired volumes; or breath frequency. There is also a two minute alarm silence button.

Comment

The Servo 900C does not have quite the degree of sophistication of some of the newer machines, but it is relatively simple to use, has adequate alarms, and has proved very reliable. It has consequently been a popular choice for both adult and paediatric use. Patient cycling was associated with an unacceptably high impedance to respiration in the 900B model, but this defect has been cured in later models.[8 9]

In the latest Servo 300 range of ventilators the control and monitoring panel has been separated from the main drive unit. The machine uses dedicated supply modules for oxygen and air, and as each module can supply a range of flows from 6 ml/min to 180 l/min the machine is suitable for neonatal, paediatric, or adult use. The ventilator can be flow triggered, and conversion from one size of patient to another is effected by a switch that automatically adjusts the triggering and monitoring functions to suit the patient. There are some additional modes, such as volume support and pressure controlled SIMV breaths. The setting up procedure for each mode is simplified by the "set parameter guide" in which lights appear sequentially by each control to indicate which control should be set for the chosen mode. Both the Servo 900 and 300 ventilators provide outputs for feeding data into computer operated patient management systems.

Hamilton Veolar

The Hamilton Veolar is designed to be used with oxygen-air mixtures only. The machine consists of a pneumatic system and an electronic control system. It requires a supply of medical grade compressed air and oxygen at a pressure of 3.5 bar (50 psi), though it will function satisfactorily with input pressures ranging from 2 to 8 bar (29–116 psi). The gas pressures are reduced to 1.5 bar (22 psi) by precision regulators, and the flows metered by two valves which also control the oxygen concentration. The gases then pass into an aluminium reservoir which holds almost 8 l of gas at a pressure of 350 cm H_2O. A safety valve blows off if the tank pressure exceeds 400 cm H_2O.

The mixed gas flows to the patient through an electronically controlled inspiratory valve which generates the required flow pattern. An oxygen analyser, safety ambient air inlet valve, and overpressure safety valve are situated between the flow control valve and the patient; a large, electronically controlled expiratory valve is situated on the bottom of the machine. Airway pressure, flow, and volume are derived from a variable orifice flow meter situated at the patient Y piece, but in the event of malfunction the microprocessor will switch to internal sensors.

The disposable flow meter head has a dead space of 9 ml and consists of a diaphragm with a small hinged flap which opens progressively as flow is increased (see fig 3.12). The flap is cut with great precision and is designed so that the pressure drop across the diaphragm is linearly related to flow rate. The pressure sensing lines are continually flushed by a low flow of gas to prevent blockage. There are two microprocessor systems which check each other. One interprets the signals from the front panel controls and generates all the displays and alarms and the other controls the servomechanisms activating the inspiratory and expiratory valves.

Controls

The front panel is divided into three parts: the control panel along the bottom, the monitoring panel at the top left, and the alarm panel at the top right (fig 6.3). The controls are simple to operate. A choice of mode is first made by pressing one of five buttons on the left of the control panel. These offer controlled or synchronised mechanical ventilation (the assist-control mode); SIMV; spontaneous ventilation (CPAP and inspiratory pressure support); MMV (here termed minimum minute ventilation); and pressure controlled ventilation.

Flow generator mode. The control knobs for CMV lie to the right of the mode selection buttons. There is a dual control knob for CMV and SIMV frequency, a tidal volume control, and a dual control for inspiratory and expiratory phases expressed as a percentage of total cycle time. The design of the dual control for inspiratory and expiratory phases is, at first, somewhat confusing because the expiratory knob must first be set to the point in the cycle at which the operator wishes expiration to start. The inspiratory knob is then set to the point where inspiration should stop. The pause time is the difference between the position of the pointers on the inspiratory and expiratory controls. If these are contiguous there is no pause. The advantage of this arrangement is that the position of the pointer on the expiratory knob then indicates the I:E ratio on the background scale. To the far right is a control for selection of one of seven flow waveforms. The settings on these five controls determine the pattern of the mandatory breath.

Inspiratory flow rate can be displayed on the patient monitor, or calculated from the tidal volume and duration of inspiration if constant flow is used. For a given tidal volume and inspiratory time, peak flow with either of the ramp waveforms would be twice that of the constant flow waveform, and peak flow with a sine wave would be 1.57 times that of the constant flow waveform.

Underneath the CMV section are the controls for trigger sensitivity (automatically compensated for PEEP/CPAP), a dual control for PEEP/CPAP and inspiratory pressure support levels, and controls for $O_2\%$ and the flow trigger sensitivity. There are also push buttons for initiation of a mandatory breath, an oxygen flush, and a controlled period of medication for nebuliser gas flow. The nebuliser function may be modified to control the concentration of nitric oxide delivered to the patient's airway, should this be required. (Nitric oxide is a pulmonary vasodilator which may be administered by inhalation in concentrations of 10–40 parts per million to patients with severe ARDS. Low concentrations seem to increase blood flow to

136

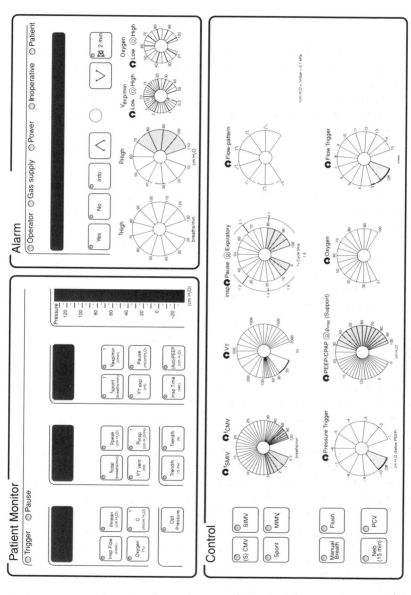

Fig 6.3 Hamilton Veolar control panel (by courtesy Hamilton Medical, Hamilton GB Ltd, Kimpton Link Business Centre, Kimpton Road, Sutton, Surrey, SM3 9QP).

ventilated areas of lung, so increasing arterial PO_2, while higher concentrations may reduce pulmonary artery pressure without affecting systemic vascular resistance. The value of this form of therapy is still under investigation.)

Pressure generator mode. In the pressure generator mode the ventilator is servocontrolled to produce a constant inspiratory pressure, inspiration being time or patient cycled. The mode is selected by pressing the PCV (pressure controlled ventilation) button and then setting the frequency and inspiratory and expiratory time controls. The choice of time or patient cycling and inflation pressure is set with the yes/no and up/down arrow buttons on the alarm display panel.

Other modes. The factors controlling the mandatory breaths have been detailed above. The ventilator may be pressure or flow triggered to produce a CMV breath with each inspiration, the sensitivity being adjusted by the appropriate control on the left or right of the control panel. With these modes there is a 0.2 second period at the beginning of expiration during which the ventilator will not respond to the trigger mechanism in order to prevent "stacking" of breaths.

Both airway pressure and flow are sensed from the pneumotachograph unit at the patient Y piece, thus minimising the trigger delay. When the flow trigger is engaged the ventilator generates a bias flow through the patient tubing which matches the flow sensitivity selected. This flow supplies the initial demand from the patient, thus minimising the work of breathing before the trigger is activated. The bias flow ceases at the end of inspiration, so that there is no impedance to expiration, but is gradually re-established during expiration as the patient's expiratory flow declines.

The ventilator performs as a demand flow system when in the spontaneous mode and requires adjustment of the pressure or flow trigger sensitivity, CPAP level, pressure support level (if required), and O_2 concentration. With spontaneous breathing modes it is possible to activate a special backup mechanism that provides mechanical ventilation in the event of apnoea.

Inspiratory pressure support may be provided during the spontaneous breathing mode and SIMV. With SIMV, synchronisation of a mandatory breath with a spontaneous breath will occur if the patient makes an inspiratory effort during a synchronisation "window." In the SIMV mode the CMV controls are first set to define the tidal volume, frequency, and inspiratory-expiratory times of the mandatory breaths. (An end inspiratory pause is not well tolerated when the breathing is assisted.) The duration of the SIMV window in seconds is then 60/CMV frequency. The SIMV frequency control is then set to extend the expiratory time to allow the patient to take spontaneous breaths between the mandatory breaths, the time between beginning of each SIMV window in seconds being 60/SIMV frequency. For example, if the CMV frequency is 15 breaths/min and the SIMV frequency 6 breaths/min, the window will last for 4 seconds and will occur at 10 second intervals. If the ventilator is not triggered during this period it will deliver a mandatory breath at the end of the window.

The MMV mode on this machine is more sophisticated than on some others. It is a spontaneous breathing mode with pressure support, but whereas the level of support is preset by the operator in the spontaneous mode, in the MMV mode the level of support is determined by the machine. When MMV is engaged the pressure support starts at the level set on the pressure support control. The machine then measures the tidal volume and frequency over eight breaths and calculates the minute volume that would result from that pattern of breathing. This is compared with the minute volume set on the MMV control, and the level of pressure support is gradually adjusted until the desired minute volume is reached. The machine continues the process of measurement and adjustment and will reduce support if the patient increases the spontaneous minute volume. When using the MMV mode it is important to set close limits on the frequency and minute volume alarms to ensure that these variables are maintained within reasonable limits.

If apnoea occurs, alarms will sound, but no mandatory breath will be delivered unless the apnoea backup ventilation mechanism has been switched on. It is important to note that this mechanism must be switched on before the power to the machine is switched on. If the machine is in the MMV mode the mechanism will switch it into the SIMV mode. If it is in a spontaneous breathing or SIMV mode, the machine will switch to the CMV settings.

Monitors and alarms

The Hamilton Veolar is a highly versatile ventilator which has a complicated monitoring and alarm system to cope with the various modes of use. The monitor panel contains a bar graph that continuously displays airway pressure and three digital displays that enable three of the 14 measured variables to be displayed at any one time. Total thoracic compliance and inspiratory and expiratory airway resistance can be calculated and displayed if a constant flow pattern with end inspiratory pause is being used, and there are a number of sophisticated trend displays. The monitoring system may be extended by connecting it to an additional display unit with dedicated software (Leonardo), which provides facilities for complete data acquisition, real time display of wave forms, X/Y plots, and trends for up to 21 days. The alarm panel contains a 31 character alphanumeric display for alarm messages; controls to set the alarm ranges for breathing frequency, airway pressure, expired volume, and oxygen concentration; and other LED alarm indicators. It also has a 2 minute alarm silence button to cover procedures such as tracheal tube suction.

139

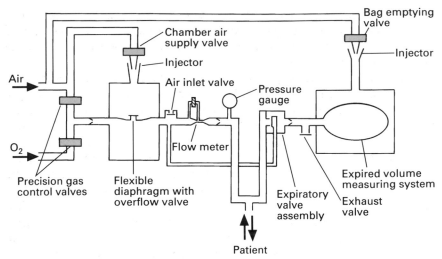

Fig 6.4   Engström Elvira pneumatic system.

Comment

The Hamilton Veolar is an innovative ventilator which has the advantage that the work of breathing and triggering delay is minimised by the provision of a bias flow and the measurement of both pressure and flow close to the patient. Tidal volume is also measured at this point, so obviating errors due to the internal compliance of the breathing system.

The Hamilton Amadeus ventilator has been designed to provide a less costly alternative to the Veolar with the same pneumatic specification. The monitoring has been reduced to a single switched display, and the alphanumeric alarm display has been replaced by simple indicating alarms. The MMV mode, optional pressure sensor, and nebuliser are not provided as standard.

Engström Elvira

The first Engström ventilator, the 200, was described in 1954.[9] Its successor, the 300, which was introduced in 1968, utilised the same mechanical principles but had an autoclavable patient circuit. The Engström Erica was the first microprocessor controlled Engström ventilator and has now been replaced by the Elvira; it uses a similar pneumatic concept but has an improved spontaneous breathing and triggering system, together with inbuilt facilities for gas exchange and metabolic monitoring.

The concentration of oxygen in air is controlled by precision needle valves, which ensure that the concentration is not affected by back pressure, and the mixture is then fed into a reservoir which is divided into two by a flexible diaphragm (fig 6.4). The volume of gas in this reservoir is regulated by an

140

electronically controlled inlet valve. In the event of power failure this valve remains open, thus ensuring that the patient continues to receive a supply of fresh gas. The reservoir is also fitted with a mechanical valve that opens if the reservoir becomes overfilled.

The breath pattern is generated by compressing the diaphragm with compressed air, the pattern of airflow being controlled electronically by a precision valve and amplified by an injector. The flow and pressure of the gas leaving the reservoir is monitored by a venturi type of flow sensor, and a pressure transducer controls the inspiratory pressure and CPAP level. A second pressure sensor measures the pressure in the inspiratory limb of the breathing system. Since the maximum flow rate of gas mixture through the filler valve is 0.5 l/sec and the chamber has a volume of 1.5 l, the patient can draw a maximum of 2 l gas from the chamber in any one second (120 l/min). If this value is exceeded an air inlet valve opens, diluting the inspired gas.

The expiration port is closed by a balloon valve that is connected to the mixed gas reservoir and so is closed when the reservoir pressure is increased during inspiration. During expiration the reservoir pressure falls and the valve opens. When PEEP is applied the pressure in the reservoir and the balloon is maintained by continued flow through the precision valve and injector. Expired volume is measured by directing the expired gas into a bag contained in a rigid chamber. The bag is emptied during inspiration by injecting a known flow of gas into the chamber outside the bag, and the time taken to empty the bag is recorded by a pressure transducer in the chamber. This unique system eliminates the problems of calibrating flow meters for variations in expired gas composition.

Controls

The front panel is divided into four sections (fig 6.5). The upper section contains an analogue display of airway pressure on the left and a luminescent screen on the right. The left portion of the luminescent screen always provides a digital display of expired minute volume, tidal volume, oxygen (%), and I:E ratio. The right side of the screen displays digital and analogue data (such as the airway pressure trace) selected by the user; these may be displaced by alarm messages.

The section below these displays contains the controls to set the alarm limits for minute volume, airway pressure, and spontaneous breathing rate, together with reset and alarm silence buttons; the bottom two sections contain the ventilator controls.

Flow generator mode. After setting the tidal volume and frequency controls it is necessary to choose between the ascending or descending ramp and constant flow waveforms and then to set the flow rate and inspiratory plateau time. Since these three parameters determine the duration of inspiration, the choice of values is greatly helped by reference to the I:E ratio display.

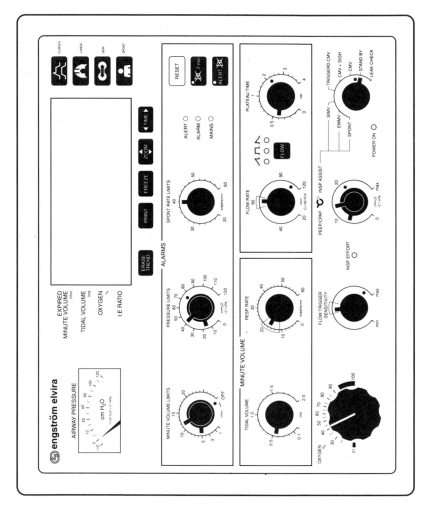

Fig 6.5   Engström Elvira control panel (by courtesy Gambro Engström AB, S161 02 Bromma, Sweden and Engström MIE Ltd, Falcon Road, Sowton Industrial Estate, Exeter EX2 7NA, Devon).

The simplest way of setting these controls is to set the plateau time first. If compliance is to be computed it is necessary to have an end inspiratory pause of about 0.3 seconds to ensure equilibrium between airway and alveolar pressure. The pattern of inspiratory airflow should be selected next. As discussed in chapter 2, there is little evidence that flow patterns have any important effect on gas exchange, though gas distribution is slightly improved by a descending ramp pattern since this fills the lung early in inspiration and generates the highest mean airway pressure. An ascending ramp pattern will result in the highest peak airway pressure (since the pressure drop along the airways will be maximal when airflow peaks at end inspiration) but the lowest mean pressure. For a given tidal volume and duration of inspiration, peak flow with either of the ramp patterns will be twice that of the continuous flow pattern. There seems to be little advantage in using the ramp patterns, so most workers will elect to use the constant flow pattern, which also has the advantage that it permits continuous measurement of airway resistance.

When the pattern has been chosen, the inspiratory flow rate can be adjusted to obtain the desired I:E ratio. The I:E ratio is limited to a maximum of 5:1 and inspiratory time to 5 seconds. At the end of this period the machine will switch to expiration. If the inspiratory flow rate has been set at such a level that the tidal volume is not delivered within this time the low tidal volume alarm will sound.

Other modes. The Engström Elvira has facilities for CPAP, triggered CMV (assisted ventilation), inspiratory pressure support, SIMV, and EMMV (extended mandatory minute volume). Patient triggering is effected by the venturi flow sensor in the machine, and the sensitivity is controlled by a knob on the lower panel. It is also possible to move the airway pressure sensing tube to the patient Y piece and to use this for patient triggering. This is useful if the machine is being used with a high resistance humidifier, which would create a high work of breathing for the patient if internal flow triggering were to be used. When the external connection to the Y piece is in place the ventilator responds to either the flow trigger or to a reduction in airway pressure exceeding a rate of 3 cm H_2O/s.

Inspiratory pressure support can be used with the spontaneous, SIMV, and EMMV modes. The level of support provided can be calculated from the inspiratory assist setting minus the PEEP/CPAP level. The inspiratory pressure builds up during the inspiration, and the breath cycle is terminated by a decrease in flow below the flow sensitivity level. If the assisted breath exceeds 7 seconds, the low rate (apnoea) alarm will be activated. During SIMV the patient can trigger the ventilator only during a timing window which occupies the last 25% of each breathing cycle, the frequency of this cycle being set by the respiratory rate setting. If the patient takes a spontaneous breath outside the trigger window it will be assisted by the

143

preset level of inspiratory support. The machine measures the level of spontaneous activity outside the trigger window in terms of rate and tidal and minute volumes, but it should be noted that this excludes the breaths taken during the window.

The EMMV mode differs from the standard MMV mode in that the machine will deliver more than the set MMV should the patient's spontaneous minute volume exceed this value. Owing to difficulties in ensuring sufficient measurement accuracy at low minute volumes it is recommended that the technique should not be used with minute volumes below 2.5 l/min. The mandatory minute volume is set with the respiratory rate and tidal volume controls. The ventilator tracks the spontaneous breathing activity and supplies a mandatory breath if the patient's spontaneous activity results in a lower minute volume. This breath is not delivered during a spontaneous breath or for 0.3 seconds afterwards. There are two additional safety features. Firstly, if the patient takes a large spontaneous breath the machine imposes a maximum delay between the last spontaneous breath and the delivery of a mandatory breath. Secondly, if the inspiratory flow rate is inadvertently set at too low a level for delivery of the preset tidal volume, the machine will deliver the preset tidal volume at 10 bpm until the deficiency in volume is made up. The low tidal volume alert will also be activated.

Monitors and alarms

The monitor and alarm section of the ventilator is separate from the control section. There are audible and visual alarms for gas supplies and electrical power, and patient related alarms for oxygen concentration, expired volume, airway pressure, and breathing rate. The patient related alarms are displayed on the right side of the luminescent screen. To the right of this screen are four buttons that are used to call up specific displays. The CURVES button yields analogue displays of pressure, inspiratory flow, or CO_2 concentration (if an analyser is connected); the LUNGS button generates digital data on respiratory resistance, compliance, peak and mean airway pressures, and PEEP/CPAP levels. This data can also be displayed in trend format. The third button (GEM) displays oxygen uptake, carbon dioxide output, respiratory quotient, and metabolic rate and the fourth (SPONT), data on spontaneous respiratory activity. Again, the data can be shown in digital or trend formats. To obtain the necessary data for the metabolic measurements, it is necessary to add a CO_2 analyser with special gas sampling tube and to perform several checks and calibrations before making the measurement.

Comment

The Engström Elvira is relatively simple to use, has a prioritised and clear alarm system, and has the additional advantage that it is designed to enable metabolic monitoring to be carried out. The patient breathing system, expiratory valve, and expired gas volume measuring assembly can be removed for sterilisation.

Dräger Evita

The Dräger Evita ventilator uses servocontrolled valves on the oxygen and air lines to control both the oxygen concentration and the inspiratory flow pattern. If there is a gas supply failure, ambient air can be drawn into the breathing system. A blow off valve in the inspiratory line prevents the inflation pressure exceeding 100 cm H_2O, and an adjustable pressure limit terminates the mandatory breath when the set value is exceeded. Airway pressure is measured in both the inspiratory and expiratory lines, and expired volume is measured by a hot wire sensor at the outlet from the machine. Two ventilators may be connected together to permit synchronised independent lung ventilation.

Controls

The front panel has three sections (fig 6.6). On the left is a large luminescent display screen with buttons for ventilation mode and menu selection. The controls are situated in the bottom section on the right side and can be covered by a hinged lid. Above, there are digital displays of O_2% and expired minute volume, the latter with adjustable high/low alarm limits, and a small luminescent display for measured values. The ventilator can function as a flow or pressure generator and can be used in the spontaneous breathing (assist, CPAP, inspiratory pressure support), SIMV, and MMV modes. It can also be used for BIPAP (biphasic positive airway pressure breathing) and has facilities for the measurement of inspiratory occlusion pressure ($P_{0.1}$) and intrinsic PEEP.

Flow and pressure generator modes. These modes are selected by pressing the IPPV button above the large display screen and then adjusting the oxygen concentration, tidal volume, frequency, I:E ratio, and PEEP controls. The end inspiratory pause time is then set by adjusting the inspiratory flow rate control. In this mode depression of the "t, Vt, f, R, C" button results in the display of the measured values of inspired gas temperature, expired tidal volume, frequency, resistance, and compliance on the small luminescent screen, while the airway pressure trace is shown on the large screen. If it is desired to limit the peak pressure, the Pmax control is adjusted to a pressure about 3 cm above the plateau pressure (pressure limited ventilation). This automatically sets the high airway pressure alarm to a value 10 mbar above Pmax. If the "Paw" button below the small display is pressed, it will display the maximum, plateau, PEEP, and mean pressures. To obtain pressure

145

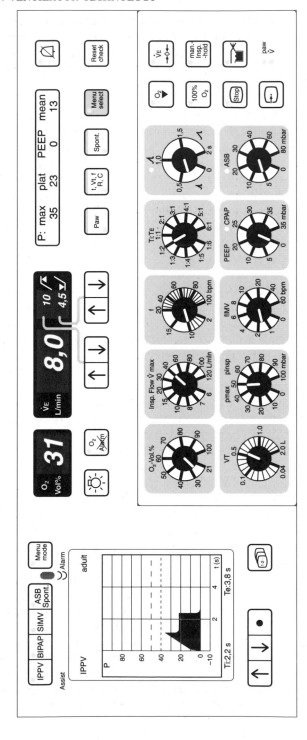

Fig 6.6 Dräger Evita 2 display and control panel (by courtesy Drägerwerk AG, Moislinger Allee 53/55, 23542 Lübeck, Germany).

controlled ventilation (for example, when it is desirable to compensate for a small leak around the tracheal tube), the tidal volume must be increased until the measured expired volume is adequate. By increasing the inspiratory flow rate it is possible to produce an approximately square wave of pressure so that the ventilator behaves as a constant pressure generator.

Other modes. Assisted breathing can be produced by activating the patient trigger control. Each triggered breath will then be indicated by the green diode to the upper left of the large display screen. Spontaneous breathing with CPAP can be engaged by pressing the "ASB/Spont" button above the large display and then adjusting the PEEP/CPAP control to the appropriate level. In all the spontaneous breathing modes (SIMV, MMV, CPAP/ASB, and BIPAP) the small luminescent display shows the spontaneous minute volume and frequency, together with the CPAP level, when the "spont" button below the display is pressed. In the Evita 1, inspiratory pressure support (labelled assisted spontaneous breathing or ASB) can be added by manipulation of the "intermittent PEEP/ASB" control, which controls the inspiratory support pressure. In addition, the rate of pressurisation can be varied by manipulation of the trigger control knob. In the Evita 2 the two controls are in a similar position but the lower control is dedicated to ASB only. In this mode an adjustable, flow sensitive trigger (1–15 l/min) can be brought into action by using the menu function.

SIMV is selected by pressing the button above the large display screen, and the SIMV frequency is set with the IMV frequency control, the pattern of the mandatory breath being determined by the IPPV settings of tidal volume, frequency, and inspiration:expiration ratio. The duration of the trigger window is 5 seconds, and the trigger sensitivity is automatically set to 0.7 cm H_2O below the CPAP/PEEP level. In the original model of the Evita, MMV was also selected by a button above the large display and the desired volume set on the tidal volume and IMV frequency controls. In the Evita 2, however, it is selected by use of the menu button, and the controls are then set in the same manner. Extra mandatory breaths are supplied when the spontaneous component becomes inadequate, and the "t, Vt, f, R, C" and "Paw" buttons may be used to display the mandatory and spontaneous components of respiration on the small luminescent screen.

The BIPAP mode permits the patient to breathe spontaneously at alternating high and low CPAP levels. In the Evita 1 the high and low times were adjusted by using the large display screen menu. In the Evita 2 the mode is selected by pressing the button above the large display and the settings are controlled by using the inspiratory pressure control knob ("Pinsp") to set the high pressure and the CPAP control to set the lower pressure. The frequency and inspiratory:expiratory ratio controls must also be adjusted to set the appropriate durations of high and low pressure. These are automatically synchronised with the patient's spontaneous respiratory activity. The periods at high and low pressure may be adjusted to create a ventilatory pattern similar to that imposed by CMV, or may be alternated at much slower frequencies. It is claimed that the spontaneous breathing component minimises the mean intrathoracic pressure and reduces the need for sedation, while CO_2 clearance is maintained by the regular alteration in lung volume.

The menu functions include tachypnoea monitoring, apnoea monitoring during CPAP/ASB (which enables the machine to switch over to IPPV when apnoea occurs), and the measurement of intrinsic PEEP and occlusion pressure. Intrinsic PEEP is measured by closing both inspiratory and expiratory valves at the end of a normal expiration and holding them closed for the duration of the next inspiration. During this period, pressure equilibrium between the lung and the breathing system occurs. The equilibrium pressure is then compared with the PEEP level to calculate the intrinsic PEEP.

The occlusion pressure ($P_{0.1}$) is the pressure generated against a closed airway during the first 0.1 seconds of a spontaneous inspiration; it is generally considered to provide a good index of neural respiratory drive. In the Evita the measurement is initiated when the spontaneous inspiration has caused the airway pressure to decrease to -0.5 mbar and is terminated by opening of the inspiratory valve 100 msec later. Since the rate of decrease of pressure after occlusion may be affected by expansion of the volume of gas between the valve and patient, this should be minimised by excluding large volume humidifiers from the breathing system during the period of measurement.

Monitors and alarms

The screen displays of the monitored variables are comprehensive. There are additional facilities for monitoring specific modalities – for example, tachypnoea during SIMV, MMV, and IPS.

Comment

The Dräger Evita is a versatile ventilator with a large screen display of airway pressure or flow pattern. Status reports providing the relevant information concerning a particular ventilation mode are also displayed on this screen. The Evita 1 was the first ventilator to include the BIPAP mode. The Evita 2 has an extended range and may now be used for paediatric or adult patients. It also has an improved, autoclavable expiratory valve assembly.

Puritan Bennett 7200 series

With the exception of the rotary control knob for setting the PEEP level, the Puritan Bennett ventilator is controlled entirely by a keyboard, which

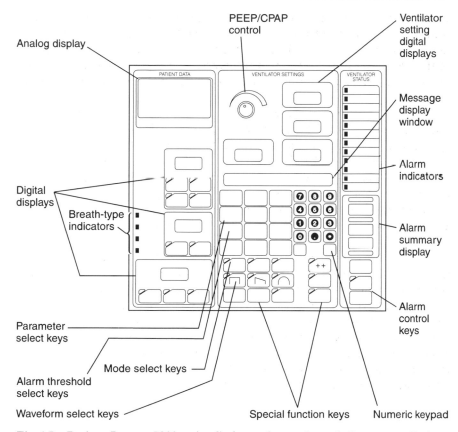

Fig 6.7   Puritan Bennett 7200 series display and control panel (by courtesy Puritan Bennett, Unit 1, Heathrow Causeway Estate, 152–176 Great South West Road, Hounslow, Middlesex TW4 6JS).

may be of the standard or enhanced pattern (fig 6.7). When the ventilator is switched on it runs a "power on" self test, and if this is satisfactory it initiates ventilation using the last entered values. Ventilator settings may be changed by pressing a ventilator setting key and keying in the desired value. The "enter" button is then pressed. If the setting is within the appropriate range the ventilator bleeps twice; if it is outside acceptable limits the ventilator bleeps four times and displays the message, "invalid entry."

The ventilator mixes air and oxygen by using rapidly acting solenoid valves controlled by the microprocessor. These valves also control the flow profile. CMV is set by adjusting the values for tidal volume, respiratory frequency, peak flow, and inspiratory plateau time. The inspiratory time is a function of tidal volume, flow pattern, and peak flow rate; expiratory time is the total cycle time minus the sum of inspiratory and plateau times. Since an

149

ascending or descending ramp flow pattern requires double the flow rate, and a sine wave pattern 1.57 times that of a constant pattern of flow, in order to generate the same tidal volume in the same time, it can be seen that the operator requires more than the usual skill in selecting the appropriate values for each of the variables. For this reason the sophisticated monitoring panel displays all the variables of the selected pattern and warns if, for example, the I:E ratio is outside the physiological range.

In the CMV mode PEEP can be applied or a sigh pattern keyed in. The ventilator can also be used in the pressure limited mode. Assisted breathing can be used by adjusting the trigger sensitivity and this can be combined with an apnoea alarm and backup CMV. Inspiratory pressure support may be provided in the assist mode, inspiration being terminated when the inspiratory flow rate falls to 5 l/min, when the airway pressure is more than 1.5 cm H_2O above the sum of PEEP plus inspiratory support level, or when inspiration lasts more than 5 seconds. SIMV and CPAP are available. The PEEP valve is unusual in that it is activated by a flow of gas from a venturi which is directed to the rear side of the expiratory valve diaphragm.

One of the unique features of this machine is a completely separate backup ventilation system with preset conditions which comes into play automatically when the ventilator detects an abnormality in the control microprocessor or power source. Another is the flow-by option, which provides a very sensitive method of triggering the ventilator.[10, 11] A continuous gas flow of 5–6 l/min is passed round the breathing system and the ventilator triggered by a reduction in this baseline flow when the patient breathes in. The sensitivity of the trigger can be adjusted by changing the flow sensitivity, which is normally set to about half the base flow rate. Flow-by will not work when the nebuliser is being used and requires careful adjustment to get the optimum results.

Comment

The Puritan Bennett is a highly sophisticated ventilator which has many facilities and a highly complex monitoring and alarm system. Setting the controls poses no problem to the computer literate younger generation but may initially prove time consuming for those used to more conventional control systems.

Summary

The differences in the setting up procedures required for these ventilators are summarised in table 6.2 (p 130).

In the CMV mode the Servo ventilator requires adjustment of the minute volume, frequency, and inspiratory and pause times. The ventilator will then adjust the peak flow with either of the two flow waveforms to ensure that the correct tidal volume is delivered. With the Hamilton Veolar it is necessary to set tidal rather than minute volume, but the flow pattern is again the result of the other settings. In the Engström Elvira and Dräger Evita the primary settings are tidal volume, frequency, inspiratory:expiratory ratio, and peak flow, so that the pause time becomes the dependent variable; in the Puritan Bennett 7200 series the dependent variable is the inspiratory time. Since the operator is usually unaware of the relation between the peak flow rate and waveform shape (for example, that the peak flow with a sine wave needs to be 1.57 times that with a square wave flow pattern to deliver the same tidal volume in the same inspiratory time), it is necessary to provide an alarm system to warn the operator that the setting is incompatible with a safe inspiratory:expiratory ratio.

Although all these ventilators have proved satisfactory in use, most intensive care units will tend to use one make, so that nursing and medical staff can become familiar with the controls and monitors. Microprocessor technology makes it easy to adapt all these machines to encompass new ventilatory modes, but since there is no clear evidence that any one mode is superior to another it would also seem wise to restrict the number of modes used to ensure that staff are familiar with the problems of patient care and monitoring that are specific to each mode.

1 Kirby RR, Banner MJ, Downs JB. *Clinical applications of ventilatory support.* Edinburgh: Churchill Livingstone, 1990.
2 Dupuis YG. *Ventilators: Theory and clinical application.* Toronto: Mosby, 1986.
3 Spearman CB, Sanders HG. The new generation of mechanical ventilators. *Resp Care* 1987;**32**:403–14.
4 Bersten AD, Skowronski GA, Oh TE. New generation ventilators. *Anaesth Intensive Care* 1986;**14**:293–305.
5 Kacmarek RM, Meklaus GJ. The new generation of mechanical ventilators. *Crit Care Clin* 1990;**6**:551–78.
6 Hayes B. Ventilators: a current assessment. In: Atkinson RS, Adams AP, eds. *Recent advances in anaesthesia and analgesia.* Edinburgh: Churchill Livingstone, 1994:83–101.
7 Tobin MJ. *Principles and practice of mechanical ventilation.* New York: McGraw-Hill, 1994.
8 Ingelstedt S, Jonson B, Nordström L, Olsson S-G. On automatic ventilation. Part 1: A servo-controlled ventilator measuring expired minute volume, airway flow and pressure. *Acta Anaesthesiol Scand* 1972;(Suppl 47):7–27.
9 Engström C-G. Treatment of severe cases of respiratory paralysis by the Engström universal respirator. *BMJ* 1954;**ii**:666–9.
10 Cox D, Tinloi SF, Farrimond JG. Investigation of the spontaneous modes of breathing of different ventilators. *Intensive Care Med* 1988;**14**:532–7.
11 Samodelov LF, Falke KJ. Total inspiratory work with modern demand valve devices compared to continuous flow CPAP. *Intensive Care Med* 1988;**14**:632–9.

7 Respiratory failure: conservative treatment and indications for respiratory support

One of the major difficulties in caring for patients with respiratory problems is to decide when to intervene and provide some form of assistance to ventilation. In the patient with acute lung disease the decision is based on the patient's general condition, on the ability to clear secretions by coughing, and on the blood gas levels. In the subject with a severe pre-existing impairment of lung fuction, however, it is important to assess whether the underlying disease will prevent weaning from the ventilator after the resolution of the acute episode. In such circumstances, providing mechanical assistance not only wastes resources but also causes unnecessary distress to the patient and the relatives. Although modern non-invasive methods of assisting ventilation are being used increasingly to provide respiratory support for patients with chronic conditions, it is important to evaluate each case on its merits so that scarce resources are used to best effect.

This chapter deals with the causes of respiratory failure, the basic principles of conservative treatment, and the indications for providing more active forms of respiratory support.

Respiratory failure

The main indication for mechanical assistance to ventilation is respiratory failure. Although physical signs such as cyanosis, dyspnoea, and the use of the accessory muscles of breathing are often seen in patients with respiratory failure, they are not diagnostic of the condition. The only way in which the diagnosis of respiratory failure can be made is by blood gas analysis. Respiratory failure is defined as an arterial PCO_2 greater than 6.7 kPa (50 mm Hg) or an arterial PO_2 less than 8 kPa (60 mm Hg) in a patient breathing air, at sea level, in the absence of any change in the non-respiratory component of acid-base balance.

The definition is rather prolix because it must encompass several variables.

152

For example, although the normal range ($\pm 95\%$) of arterial PCO_2 values is 4.8–5.9 kPa (36–44 mm Hg), a higher upper limit is taken to allow for sampling, storage, or analysis errors. Arterial PO_2 also varies because of airway closure in infancy and in those over the age of 40. Arterial PO_2 is approximately 9.3 kPa (70 mm Hg) at birth, increases towards normal values during the first few years of life, reaches a maximum of 13.3 kPa (100 mm Hg) in adolescence, and then declines gradually with increasing age, reaching a value of about 10.7 kPa (80 mm Hg) in those over 70 years old. These changes, and the effects of altitude and oxygen therapy, must be allowed for in the definition. The caveat concerning the state of the non-respiratory component of acid-base balance is to ensure that a compensatory increase in PCO_2 in response to a non-respiratory alkalosis is not diagnosed as ventilatory failure. This mistake has been made more than once by those who customarily look at the laboratory results rather than the patient.

Types of respiratory failure

There are basically two types of respiratory failure: ventilatory, due to a failure to match the ventilation to the CO_2 production; and hypoxaemic, due to processes that impair oxygen transfer in the lung.

Types of respiratory failure

Ventilatory
Caused by:
   Decreased alveolar ventilation due to:
      Decreased total ventilation
      Increased dead space
Results in:
   Increased alveolar and arterial PCO_2
   Decreased alveolar and arterial PO_2

Hypoxaemic
Caused by:
   Impaired oxygen transfer in lung due to:
      Ventilation/perfusion inequalities
      Intrapulmonary shunt
      Hypoxaemia increased by decreased mixed venous (PO_2)
Results in:
   Normal or decreased alveolar and arterial PCO_2
   Normal or increased alveolar PO_2
   Decreased arterial PO_2

Ventilatory failure

The arterial PCO_2 is determined by the CO_2 production and the alveolar ventilation:

$$\text{Arterial } PCO_2 \text{ (kPa)} = \frac{CO_2 \text{ production (ml/min STPD)}}{\text{alveolar ventilation (l/min BTPS)}} \times 0.115$$

The factor 0.115 is required to correct for the units of measurement. (If PCO_2 is in mm Hg the factor is 0.863.) The relation is shown in figure 2.15. As the alveolar ventilation is determined by the total ventilation and the dead space, ventilatory failure may be caused either by conditions that decrease total ventilation (respiratory centre depression, various forms of neuromuscular failure) or by conditions that make ventilation less efficient by increasing the ratio of dead space to tidal volume (pulmonary embolus, hypovolaemic shock, acute or chronic lung disease). In many patients several causes are present.

When the patient is breathing air the increase in alveolar and arterial PCO_2 decreases the alveolar and arterial PO_2. The relation is affected to a small extent by the shrinkage of alveolar gas volume resulting from the unequal exchange of CO_2 and O_2, but for clinical purposes sufficient accuracy is obtained by calculating alveolar PO_2 from the simplified form of the alveolar air equation:

alveolar PO_2 = inspired PO_2 − alveolar PCO_2/R

where R = the respiratory exchange ratio (normally 0.8). In a lung with ventilation-perfusion inequalities there will be a variation in alveolar PCO_2 between individual alveoli, so there is no one value that can be inserted into the equation. Since arterial PCO_2 is considered to represent the best measure of the average PCO_2 at which the lung is working, this value is substituted for alveolar PCO_2. The value derived from this calculation represents an ideal alveolar PO_2, that is, the PO_2 which would exist in all the alveoli were they perfectly ventilated and perfused under the defined conditions of inspired PO_2, ventilation, and gas exchange. Comparing the ideal value with the arterial value makes it possible to obtain a measure of the degree of impairment of oxygen exchange. A similar form of analysis can be applied to the determination of the different components of dead space (fig 7.1).

For a normal person breathing air:

alveolar PO_2 = 20 − 5.3/0.8 = 13.3 kPa (or 150 − 40/0.8 = 100 mm Hg)

If the PCO_2 is doubled the alveolar PO_2 becomes 20 − 10.6/0.8 = 6.75 kPa (or 150 − 80/0.8 = 50 mm Hg) and there will be a corresponding decrease in arterial PO_2. However, if the patient breathes 30% oxygen (PO_2 = 28.52 kPa or 214 mm Hg), the alveolar PO_2 will increase to 28.52 − 10.6/0.8 = 15.27kPa (or 214 − 80/0.8 = 114 mm Hg) so that the patient will not be hypoxaemic,

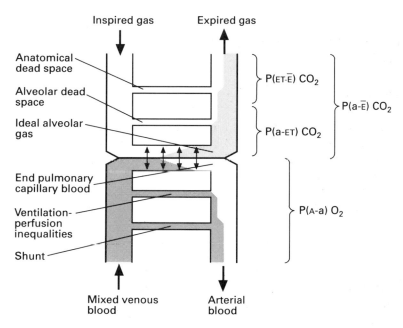

Fig 7.1 Five compartment model of lung. Gas exchange between inspired gas and mixed venous blood takes place at alveolar-capillary membrane, end pulmonary capillary blood being considered to have same composition as ideal alveolar gas. Anatomical dead space and intrapulmonary shunt compartments take no part in gas exchange. Impairments of gas exchange produced by ventilation-perfusion inequalities are quantified by equating them with alveolar dead space and venous admixture compartments. The ideal alveolar PCO_2 is assumed to be equal to the arterial PCO_2, so the presence of an alveolar dead space creates an arterial to end tidal PCO_2 difference ($P(a\text{-}ET)$ CO_2). The gas from the anatomical dead space further dilutes the mixed gas from the alveoli, so creating an end tidal to mixed expired difference ($P(ET\text{-}\bar{E})CO_2$). The sum of the two gradients ($P(a\text{-}\bar{E})CO_2$) indicates the size of the physiological dead space. Similarly, the ideal alveolar to arterial PO_2 difference ($P(A\text{-}a)O_2$) is indicative of the total venous admixture. The venous admixture effect due to ventilation-perfusion inequalities can be abolished by the breathing of a high inspired oxygen concentration (since this oxygenates blood leaving such alveoli), so that the remaining $P(A\text{-}a)O_2$ is entirely due to the presence of a right to left shunt.

even though the alveolar ventilation has been halved. Thus, adding oxygen to the inspired gas mixture will prevent arterial hypoxaemia in a patient with ventilatory failure. Indeed, if the lungs have been washed out with oxygen and the patient becomes apnoeic, aventilatory mass transfer of oxygen from the oxygen source to the pulmonary capillary blood will occur and the arterial blood will remain fully saturated for a prolonged period.

Figure 7.2 shows the relation between alveolar PCO_2 and alveolar PO_2. It may be seen that any increase in the alveolar PCO_2 results in a proportional reduction of the alveolar PO_2, the slope of the line being determined by the respiratory exchange ratio. It will be apparent that any change in the slope of

155

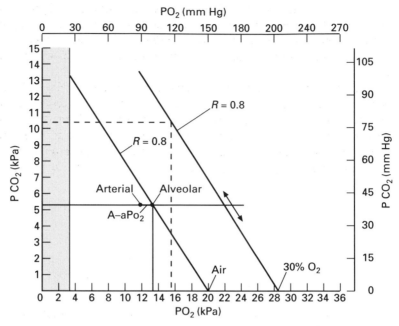

Fig 7.2 PO₂/PCO₂ diagram illustrating relation between alveolar PCO₂ and alveolar PO₂ when patient is breathing air (inspired PO₂ 20 kPa (150 mm Hg)) and 30% oxygen (inspired PO₂ 28.5 kPa (214 mm Hg)). Slope of lines depends on respiratory exchange ratio, here assumed to be 0.8. Arterial PO₂ is always less than alveolar PO₂, magnitude of alveolar-arterial PO₂ difference depending on percentage venous admixture, mixed venous oxygen content, and slope of oxygen dissociation curve. Shaded area at left represents range of arterial oxygen tensions normally incompatible with prolonged survival.

the R line will alter the relation between these two variables, and that any given increment in inspired PO_2 will produce an identical increase in the ideal alveolar PO_2Q. (However, as noted below, the increase in arterial PO_2 may be less than the increase in alveolar PO_2 because the alveolar-arterial PO_2 difference resulting from a given degree of venous admixture increases with increasing inspired PO_2, due to the shape of the oxyhaemoglobin dissociation curve.)

Hypoxaemic failure

The above calculations assumed that there was no impairment of oxygen transfer within the lungs, so that arterial PO_2 equalled alveolar PO_2. However, in patients with normal lungs there is always a small degree of ventilation-perfusion inequality due to the gravitational distribution of pulmonary blood flow, and this, together with a small component of venous admixture due to intrapulmonary shunt, causes the arterial PO_2 to be about

156

0.7–1.3 kPa (5–10 mm Hg) less than the calculated alveolar PO_2 when the patient is breathing air. Because of the flattening of the oxyhaemoglobin dissocation curve at higher PO_2 levels, this difference increases with increasing oxygen concentration and is approximately doubled when the subject is breathing 100% oxygen.

In patients with lung disease the alveolar to arterial PO_2 difference increases because of ventilation-perfusion inequalities and intrapulmonary shunts, the contribution from each of these components depending on the type of lung disease present. The mechanism by which intrapulmonary shunts cause hypoxaemia is simple to understand, for the arterial oxygen content is determined by the proportion of the total pulmonary blood flow

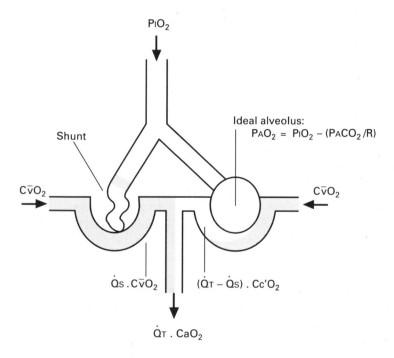

$$\dot{Q}_T \cdot CaO_2 = (\dot{Q}_T - \dot{Q}_S) \cdot C\bar{v}O_2 + (Cc'O_2 + \dot{Q}_S) \, C\bar{v}O_2$$

$$\text{or} \quad \frac{\dot{Q}_S}{\dot{Q}_T} = \frac{Cc'O_2 - CaO_2}{Cc'O_2 - C\bar{v}O_2}$$

Fig 7.3 Arterial oxygen content (CaO_2) depends on end pulmonary capillary oxygen content ($Cc'O_2$) of blood leaving ventilated lung, oxygen content of mixed venous blood ($C\bar{v}O_2$), and proportion of cardiac output ($\dot{Q}_T$) flowing through shunt ($\dot{Q}_S$). Arterial and mixed venous contents can be measured directly or calculated from PO_2, pH, and Hb; $Cc'O_2$ is calculated from ideal alveolar PO_2 (PAO_2) and arterial pH and Hb. The equations show how the fraction of blood passing through the shunt ($\dot{Q}_S/\dot{Q}_T$) can be derived from the $Cc'O_2$, CaO_2 and $C\bar{v}O_2$.

157

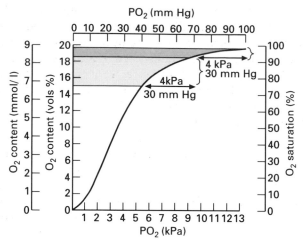

Fig 7.4 Oxygen dissociation curve to show relation between PO₂, percentage saturation, and oxygen content. Differences in oxygen content resulting from alveolar-arterial PO₂ difference of 4 kPa (30 mm Hg) at two different levels of alveolar PO₂ indicate that alveolar-arterial PO₂ difference bears little relation to magnitude of shunt.

passing through the shunt and by the oxygen contents of the oxygenated and mixed venous blood (figs 7.3 and 7.4). Hypoxaemia will be increased if the proportion of shunt increases or the mixed venous oxygen content decreases.

The mechanism by which ventilation-perfusion inequalities lead to hypoxaemia is less obvious (fig 7.5). Alveoli that are overventilated in relation to their perfusion (A′) contribute blood with a lower PCO_2 and higher PO_2 than normally ventilated and perfused alveoli (A), whereas alveoli that are

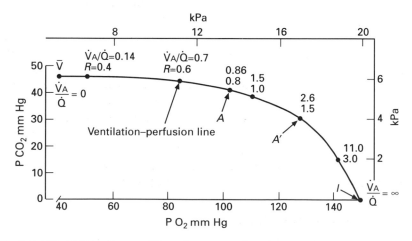

Fig 7.5 PO₂/PCO₂ diagram illustrating gas tensions in normal alveoli, and effects of variations in ventilation-perfusion ratios.

underventilated in relation to their perfusion contribute blood with a higher PCO_2 and lower PO_2 than normally ventilated and perfused alveoli. The increase in arterial PCO_2 resulting from the decreased CO_2 excretion in the underventilated alveoli stimulates the respiratory centre so that total ventilation is increased and the arterial PCO_2 is maintained at normal levels. However, the increased PO_2 in the overventilated alveoli cannot increase the saturation of the red cell beyond 100%, so that there is no mechanism for compensating for the lower PO_2 in the blood leaving the underventilated alveoli. Thus, ventilation-perfusion inequalities always result in a venous admixture effect and arterial hypoxaemia when the patient is breathing air, but CO_2 retention occurs only in the later stages of the disease when the patient is unable to sustain the high levels of total ventilation required to compensate for the reduced CO_2 excretion in the underventilated alveoli. This usually occurs when the minute volume reaches levels of about 12 l/min (see fig 2.17).

Hypoxaemia due to areas of lung with a low ventilation-perfusion ratio can be abolished by breathing concentrations of oxygen of 30-35%. However, administration of oxygen has much less effect on arterial PO_2 when hypoxaemia is due to the presence of areas of lung with no ventilation at all (intrapulmonary shunts). Under such circumstances the administration of 100% oxygen to ventilated areas of lung increases the dissolved oxygen from 3ml/l of blood to about 21 ml/l of blood. This is usually not sufficient to fully saturate the red cells coming from the areas of shunt so that hypoxaemia usually persists. Large intrapulmonary shunts may be present without there being any increase in PCO_2 because the higher level of CO_2 in the venous blood flowing through the shunt stimulates the respiratory centre and this increases ventilation. Indeed, in some circumstances the arterial PCO_2 may be lower than normal due to a hypoxic drive from the peripheral chemoreceptors, or to a reflex ventilatory drive from the lungs.

The decrease in arterial content resulting from hypoxaemic respiratory failure obviously reduces the transport of oxygen to the tissues, though local homoeostatic mechanisms may increase tissue blood flow to compensate for the reduced PO_2. An increased PCO_2 may also produce some degree of compensation, for it increases cardiac output by sympathetic stimulation of the heart and shifts the oxygen dissociation curve to the right, so increasing the volume of oxygen offloaded at a given mixed venous PO_2. It is therefore important to consider the cardiac output, haemoglobin concentration, and position of the oxyhaemoglobin dissociation curve as well as arterial PO_2 when deciding on treatment in a patient with hypoxaemia.

Causes of respiratory failure

Although blood gas analysis provides a practical method of diagnosing the presence, type, and severity of respiratory failure, the measurements repre-

159

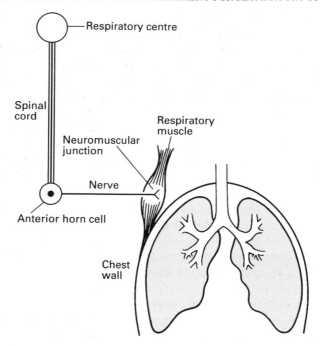

Fig 7.6 Causes of respiratory failure. Drive originates in respiratory centre and is transmitted through spinal cord, nerves, and neuromuscular junction to respiratory muscles, which act on chest wall. Inspiratory muscle forces are opposed by elastic recoil of lungs and by airway resistance.

sent only the end stage of complex patterns of failure of different components of the respiratory system. The next section deals primarily with the causes of ventilatory failure, but this is often complicated by pre-existing lung disease, the presence of infection, or effects produced by the retention of secretions. For this reason the term respiratory failure has been retained. Figure 7.6 summarises the causes of respiratory failure and shows that it results either from a failure to generate an adequate contraction of the respiratory muscles or from the development of increased impedances to the expansion of the lungs. These factors are best considered by following the neuromuscular pathway from the respiratory centre to the periphery.[1]

Factors influencing the generation of muscle force

Respiratory centre. The central drive to respiration originates in the respiratory centre in the medulla. Neural output is predominantly governed by the central chemoreceptors, but the centre also receives afferent information from the peripheral chemoreceptors, the reticular activating system, and the cortex. Lesions affecting these areas or connecting pathways can therefore result in a decrease in neural drive. Common causes of central respiratory depression are a reduced blood supply to the respiratory centre (hypotension or cardiac arrest), trauma, compression due to raised intra-cranial pressure, and various forms of encephalitis. Poliomyelitis also affects the ventilatory nuclei in the brain stem, and sleep apnoea may result. Drug overdose (especially with the opiates) is a common cause of respiratory depression, but this may also be produced by normal doses of hypnotic, sedative, or opioid drugs if these are given to patients who already have an abnormality of central respiratory control. There are also patients who have normal ventilation when awake but develop apnoea when the cortical input is abolished during sleep. This syndrome (Ondine's curse) is usually associated with medullary infarction involving the ventilatory nuclei or their descending tracts and may be seen after surgery on the high spinal cord or brainstem.

An assessment of neural drive can be made by measuring the P_{01}, the subatmospheric pressure generated in the airway during the first 0.1 of a second after an intermittent occlusion of the airway during spontaneous breathing, but this is not easy to measure in the clinical environment. Assessing chemoreceptor sensitivity by recording ventilatory CO_2 response curves is equally difficult, and their interpretation is complicated by the approximately 16-fold difference in CO_2 sensitivity in normal subjects. One of the other problems in assessment is that sleep may reduce the input to the respiratory centre so that episodes of apnoea become apparent only when the patient is carefully observed in a controlled environment. Periods of centrally

---

Causes of respiratory failure

Inadequate inspiratory force
    Decreased central drive
    Cervical cord injury
    Spinal cord disease
    Peripheral neuropathy
    Impaired transmission at neuromuscular junction
    Muscle disease or fatigue
    Impaired transmission of force to lungs
        Flail segment of chest wall
        Ruptured diaphragm
        Pneumothorax

Increased impedances to ventilation
    Increased stiffness or distortion of chest wall
    Increased pressure below diaphragm
    Air or fluid in pleural space
    Decreased lung compliance
    Increased airways resistance

mediated sleep apnoea are particularly common when opioid analgesia is used after major surgery.[2]

Cervical cord. Spinal artery infarction, compression by tumour, or trauma to the cervical cord will result in quadriplegia and respiratory arrest if the damage is located at or above the origin of the phrenic nerves (C3–5) which supply the diaphragm. Cervical trauma below this level results in diaphragmatic breathing which is usually adequate to sustain life, though its efficiency is reduced by the concomitant paralysis of the intercostal and abdominal muscles.[3] The combination of inspiratory and expiratory muscle weakness decreases the efficiency of the cough mechanism and increases the risk of developing respiratory tract infections. Patients with lower cervical cord injury often have a vital capacity of 1.2–1.5 l immediately after injury, when the chest muscles are flaccid. However, when the stage of spinal shock passes the flaccidity is replaced by spasticity and the more rigid chest wall enables vital capacities of 2.0 l or more to be attained. As a result over 80% of patients with a lesion at or below C4 can be weaned from mechanical ventilation.[1]

Spinal cord. Most of the diseases affecting the spinal cord are progressive, and respiratory failure tends to be a terminal event. In such circumstances it is generally agreed that active treatment has little to offer. However, in some patients non-invasive techniques of respiratory support can relieve symptoms. For example, more than 50% of patients with motor neurone disease (amyotrophic lateral sclerosis) die from complications such as aspiration and pneumonia within three years of diagnosis.[1] Respiratory insufficiency is most common in the later stages, but some patients may develop respiratory symptoms early in the course of the disease or even present with respiratory failure or arrest. Many of these patients can benefit from non-invasive methods of respiratory support such as nocturnal CPAP, cuirass, or intermittent positive pressure ventilation.[4]

In many parts of the world poliomyelitis is still endemic. The virus affects the anterior horn cell and may produce paralysis in the areas supplied by the cranial or spinal nerves. It may also affect the medullary cardiorespiratory centres, producing respiratory irregularities, apnoea, or other dysautonomias. Bulbar paralysis can usually be managed by postural drainage, oral suction, and feeding by nasogastric tube, but it is sometimes necessary to isolate the lungs from the mouth by using a cuffed tracheostomy tube. Paralysis localised to the spinal nerves may be treated by a device such as a tank ventilator which generates an intermittent negative pressure around the chest, but if both bulbar and spinal nerves are involved a tracheostomy and intermittent positive pressure ventilation will be required.[5] In recent years, bouts of recurrent muscle weakness have been observed in patients who had suffered poliomyelitis many years previously. The progression of this "postpolio syndrome" seems relatively slow (it results in an average loss of

162

muscle strength of about 1% per year), but it may lead to the late onset of respiratory failure.

Peripheral nerves. Acute polyneuritis (Guillain-Barré syndrome) is the most common peripheral neuropathy causing respiratory failure. The onset of symptoms is preceded by an upper respiratory or gastrointestinal infection in about half of the cases. The disease affects a variable number of spinal nerves, the paralysis usually starting in the legs and then spreading to the arms and trunk. About 20% of patients will eventually require ventilatory assistance. The paralysis reaches a peak at 2–4 weeks and usually resolves in 3–6 weeks with appropriate treatment. However, about 15% of patients are left with residual weakness and another 5% will have relapsing episodes of demyelination. The disease also affects the autonomic system and results in rapid changes in pulse rate and blood pressure, which may be difficult to control.[6] Plasmapheresis shortens the stay in hospital and the intensive care unit if it is started within two weeks of the onset of symptoms.

Other causes of peripheral neuropathy that may lead to respiratory failure are acute intermittent porphyria, diphtheria, paralytic shellfish (saxitoxin) poisoning, systemic lupus erythematosus, polyarteritis nodosa, Lyme disease, and toxins such as thallium, lead, and triorthocresyl phosphate (TOCP).

Another syndrome that is being seen in intensive care units is critical illness polyneuropathy.[7] This is seen predominantly in elderly patients who have undergone a prolonged period of treatment for sepsis and multiorgan failure. Attempts to wean the patient from the ventilator are prolonged, there is muscle atrophy, and the reflexes are diminished. If the patient can be weaned, full recovery can occur.

Neuromuscular junction. The respiratory muscles are involved in about 10% of patients with myasthenia gravis, and mechanical assistance may be required to treat respiratory failure precipitated by intercurrent infection or surgery. Respiratory failure may also be precipitated by myasthenic or cholinergic crises. Treatment includes mechanical ventilation, plasmapheresis, corticosteroids, acetylcholinesterase inhibitors, and immunosuppressive agents. Thymectomy is usually recommended for patients with generalised myasthenia gravis and results in an improvement or remission in about 80% of patients who do not have a thymoma.

Botulism is another condition that affects the neuromuscular junction. The infection is derived from ingesting contaminated food or from surgical wound infection and results in a descending paralysis that initially affects the extraocular and bulbar muscles and often progresses to the respiratory muscles. Treatment involves elimination of unabsorbed toxin from the gut by enemas and gastric lavage, giving antitoxin and high doses of penicillin, and surgical treatment of any infected wounds. Severely affected patients may require mechanical ventilation for several months.

Poisoning by organophosphorus insecticides or nerve gases may also result in paralysis. Muscle relaxant drugs are given routinely during anaesthesia and their action may persist into the postoperative period either because of overdose, increased sensitivity to the drug (for example, non-depolarising relaxants in patients with myasthenia gravis), or failure of breakdown or excretion of the drug. For example, suxamethonium is broken down by plasma pseudocholinesterase and about one person in 2800 has a congenital deficiency of this enzyme. The action of drugs, such as pancuronium, that are excreted mainly by the kidney persists for prolonged periods in patients with renal failure. Vecuronium, which is normally excreted mainly by the liver, may also act for prolonged periods in patients with renal failure.[8] Muscle relaxants are also used therapeutically when patients with severe tetanus do not respond to conservative treatment.

In recent years it has become apparent that the long term use of muscle relaxant drugs such as pancuronium and vecuronium in mechanically ventilated patients may lead to generalised muscle weakness and atrophy.[9] Most of these patients were also receiving aminoglycosides and corticosteroids, so the aetiology may be multifactorial. In most cases the paralysis was totally reversible.

Respiratory muscles. Most myopathies do not produce significant respiratory dysfunction. However, patients with muscular dystrophy often die from respiratory failure in the second or third decade of life. If provided, support is usually limited to one of the non-invasive methods outlined in chapter 10. There are a few muscle diseases in which mechanical ventilation may be required while medical treatment is taking effect. One of these is dermatomyositis, which can affect both the respiratory and bulbar muscles. Mechanical support has proved lifesaving in such cases in children.

There is now increasing evidence that respiratory muscle fatigue may both precipitate respiratory failure and prevent weaning from the ventilator. There is also some evidence to suggest that disuse atrophy may occur if the muscles are rested completely by controlled mechanical ventilation for a prolonged period. The appropriate balance between rest and exercise of the respiratory muscles has not been determined and much further research is required to clarify this topic.[10]

Factors increasing the impedance to ventilation

Chest wall. The chest wall includes the ribs and diaphragm. Surprisingly, increased stiffness of the rib cage induced by such diseases as rheumatoid arthritis, scleroderma, or ankylosing spondylitis rarely produces respiratory failure, probably because diaphragmatic function is little affected. However, a deformity of the rib cage produced, for example, by kyphoscoliosis, or a floating area of rib cage resulting from trauma, commonly results in respiratory failure. This is probably due to the disturbance of ventilation-perfusion relationships in the underlying lung.

Pressure on the diaphragm from intra-abdominal distention, ascites, surgical packs, or abdominal binders pushes the diaphragm up into the chest and so causes basal collapse and a decrease in the functional residual capacity of the lungs. These conditions also limit diaphragmatic movement and so contribute to respiratory failure in the postoperative period. The effects are accentuated by the supine posture and obesity.

Pleural space. Fluid in the pleural space reduces lung volume and may produce gravitational effects on the mediastinum, great vessels, and heart. As the fluid is relatively non-elastic it transmits pressures generated by the movement of the chest wall to the lungs. Air, on the other hand, is easily compressed and expanded by the changes in intrathoracic pressure, so that the movements of the lung are less than those of the chest wall. A tension pneumothorax obviously creates specific problems that directly threaten survival.

Lungs. The power generated by the neuromuscular system is opposed by the elastic recoil of the lungs and chest wall and by the resistance of the airways. As with the chest wall, an increase in stiffness of the lungs (reduced compliance) is not a common cause of respiratory failure. Patients with a high airway resistance resulting from a localised obstruction in the trachea or bronchi also tend to maintain adequate alveolar ventilation despite a high work of breathing, even though the orifice may be only 4–6 mm in diameter. However, patients with an increase in resistance of the smaller airways, whether acute, as in asthma, or chronic, as in bronchitis, often develop respiratory failure during exacerbations of the disease. Again, it is probably the presence of infection and increased secretions, together with the hypoxaemia resulting from ventilation-perfusion inequalities, that precipitates the onset of failure.

Conservative treatment

The occurrence of respiratory failure is usually manifested by signs of respiratory distress such as an increase in respiratory rate, dyspnoea, activity of the accessory muscles and ala nasae, and there may be cyanosis and a depressed level of consciousness. Though these signs provide a warning that the patient is deteriorating, they are not in themselves an indication for the provision of some form of respiratory support, for the condition may well resolve if the appropriate conservative treatment is given. The three major lines of conservative treatment are the administration of oxygen, assistance with the removal of secretions, and drug therapy.

Oxygen therapy

Hypoxic patients who do not have a disorder of respiratory control are best treated initially with one of the standard disposable oxygen face masks. An oxygen flow of 5 l/min should result in an inspired concentration of 30-50%. Higher concentrations can be obtained only by using a closely fitting anaesthetic-type mask and breathing system with a high enough gas flow to prevent rebreathing. If the patient does not tolerate the disposable face mask a nasal catheter may be used. The catheter should be lubricated with local anaesthetic gel and passed until its tip lies behind the soft palate, care being taken to fix it firmly to the nose to prevent it passing into the oesophagus and stomach. The catheter may need to be switched to the opposite nostril at intervals of 3–4 hours. A flow of 3–4 l/min usually results in inspired concentrations of 30–40%. Oxygen masks often become displaced when worn at night; it may then be better to use nasal prongs, which can be retained in position more reliably even though they do not produce such high inspired concentrations as a correctly positioned face mask.

Controlled oxygen therapy. Patients with an acute exacerbation of chronic obstructive airways disease and an increase in PCO_2 will require controlled oxygen therapy while treatment with active physiotherapy, bronchodilators, diuretics, and antibiotics is taking effect. The problem is that such patients tend to develop further CO_2 retention when given oxygen, and when arterial PCO_2 levels exceed 10 kPa this leads to a decreased level of consciousness, an inability to cough, and a further deterioration in lung mechanics and gas exchange. It is not clear whether the increase in PCO_2 is due to depression of

---

Conservative methods of treatment

Oxygen therapy
   Emergency: 100%
   Routine: 30–50%
   Controlled: 24–35%

Removal of secretions
   Coughing, percussion, postural drainage, bronchoscopy, tracheostomy

Drug therpay
   Antibiotics
   Bronchodilators
   Steroids
   Respiratory stimulants
   Diuretics
   Inotropes and other cardiac drugs
   Pulmonary vasodilators

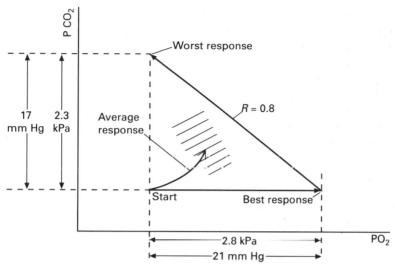

Fig 7.7 PO₂/PCO₂ diagram illustrating possible blood gas changes resulting from controlled oxygen therapy. Inspired oxygen has been increased by 3% (2.8 kPa). Ideally, arterial PO₂ should increase by a similar amount without any increase in PCO₂. The worst situation is considerable increase in PCO₂ with no increase in PO₂. Because of the slope of the PCO₂/PO₂ line (R = 0.8) the maximum increase in PCO₂ is 2.8 × 0.8 = 2.3 kPa. Usually, both arterial PO₂ and PCO₂ increase (shaded area).

the peripheral chemoreceptor hypoxic drive to respiration or to an inability of the patient to increase the minute volume to compensate for the increase in alveolar dead space induced by the increased alveolar oxygen tension. Whatever the cause, the main aim of treatment must be to relieve severe hypoxaemia while maintaining a level of consciousness that retains the patient's ability to cough and cooperate with the physiotherapist. This is done by giving carefully controlled, low concentrations of oxygen during the acute stages of the disease.

The principle of controlled oxygen therapy is that when the patient's arterial PO_2 lies on the steep part of the oxyhaemoglobin dissociation curve it requires only a small increase in inspired PO_2, and therefore in arterial PO_2, to produce a relatively large increase in arterial oxygen content and oxygen delivery. Almost invariably the increase in inspired PO_2 results in some increase in arterial PCO_2, which in turn decreases arterial PO_2, but the net effect is an increase in oxygen delivery, which helps to relieve tissue hypoxia (fig 7.7).

The simplest way of giving low concentrations of oxygen is to use a flow of 1-2 l/min with nasal prongs. This technique has the advantage that the oxygen can be given continuously and that the treatment does not interfere with eating, drinking, or coughing. However, there is a variable degree of dilution with room air, and the concentration of oxygen tends to rise as

167

ventilation decreases, thus leading to further depression of respiration and CO_2 retention.

This technique is not suitable for patients with a PCO_2 above 7–8 kPa. In these patients the oxygen concentration is best controlled by a venturi type of mask, which prevents air dilution by providing a high flow (about 40 l/min) of premixed gas with oxygen concentrations of 24%, 28%, or 35%. The patient is first given 24% oxygen and the response to treatment is then monitored by blood gas analysis. If the increase in PCO_2 during the first hour of treatment is less than 1 kPa, the inspired concentration can be increased to 28% and blood gas analysis repeated after a further hour. Usually, this level of inspired oxygen provides relief of severe hypoxaemia, but in some patients higher concentrations are required. If the increase in PCO_2 in response to 24% oxygen is more than 1 kPa or there is a decrease in conscious level, physiotherapy should be increased and the use of respiratory stimulants should be considered.

In some patients inspiratory pressure support administered by face mask may help to reduce CO_2 retention,[11] but in those with severe CO_2 retention tracheal intubation may be required. However, this should not be undertaken in those with a severe limitation of respiratory function between acute exacerbations because of the subsequent weaning difficulties.

Occasionally, a patient with a severe exacerbation may have received high concentration oxygen therapy before being admitted to hospital and may thus have developed very high PCO_2 levels. Such patients require careful evaluation before treatment is changed because any reduction in inspired oxygen concentration could result in severe hypoxaemia and death. If the patient is comatose or the PCO_2 is very high it may be necessary to control the ventilation mechanically.

Removal of secretions

Regular physiotherapy is required to encourage removal of secretions by coughing. Chest percussion, assisted coughing, and postural drainage must be performed at frequent intervals in patients with excessive secretions, particularly if the level of consciousness or cough reflex is depressed. In patients with chronic obstructive airways disease, physiotherapy must be vigorous and performed at frequent intervals; in these cases it is usually necessary for doctors and nursing staff to augment the treatments given by the physiotherapist. If a localised area of collapse does not respond to vigorous physiotherapy and postural drainage, fibreoptic bronchoscopy and suction should be used to clear secretions from the appropriate bronchus.

Drug treatment

The drugs most commonly required are antibiotics, bronchodilators, steroids, and respiratory stimulants. Diuretics will be required for the

168

treatment of pulmonary oedema, and inotropes and other drugs may be needed in patients with cardiac disease. Pulmonary vasodilators may be used in patients with pulmonary hypertension. Antibiotic treatment is usually governed by local hospital and unit policies. Patients with a tracheal tube or tracheostomy are at special risk, as are those who are immunocompromised.

The bronchodilator drugs are required in the treatment of patients with asthma and are often used in the treatment of patients with chronic obstructive airways disease, for there is often a reversible element to their airway narrowing. The selective β_2 adrenoceptor stimulants such as salbutamol and terbutaline are the safest and most effective and may be delivered by inhalation using metered doses from pressurised inhalers. In the intensive care unit they are more commonly given in the form of nebuliser solutions with gas driven nebulisers.

Patients with asthma benefit from an oxygen driven nebuliser because bronchodilator drugs tend to increase arterial hypoxaemia by decreasing hypoxic vasoconstriction in underventilated areas of lung, but in patients with an acute exacerbation of chronic obstructive airways disease the driving gas should be air or 24–28% oxygen to minimise any increase in PCO_2. It should be remembered that the dose given by nebuliser is considerably greater than that given by the pressurised inhalers (for example, 2.5 mg given over 15 minutes by nebuliser is equivalent to 25 puffs from a pressurised inhaler), so careful observation of the patient is essential.

In severe cases, drugs given by this route may be supplemented by intravenous administration. However, intravenous administration increases the incidence of side effects (tremor, headache, peripheral vasodilatation, and tachycardia). Long term treatment with these drugs may be complicated by hypokalaemia, so plasma potassium should be checked regularly.

Steroids should be given to patients with a severe attack of asthma. In adults 200 mg hydrocortisone sodium succinate may be given initially and followed by maintenance treatment. Although steroids have been used to treat acute exacerbations of obstructive airways disease, there is little objective evidence to indicate that they are of value.

Another indication for the use of a large intravenous dose of corticosteroids is as a supplement to intravenous adrenaline in treating anaphylactoid reactions to drugs. Dexamethasone has been advocated for treating brain damage due to cerebral hypoxia, and methyl prednisolone was at one time used in the treatment of septic shock. However, a recent controlled trial in patients with septic shock showed that mortality was increased in the group given corticosteroids.

There is still debate concerning the role of respiratory stimulants in patients with an acute exacerbation of chronic obstructive airways disease. Doxapram has now superseded drugs such as nikethamide, which did not produce respiratory stimulation until given in subconvulsive doses. Doxapram is given as an intravenous infusion in a dose of 1–4 mg/min, the dose being adjusted according to the patient's response. Although doxapram is undoubtedly a respiratory stimulant, it may increase oxygen consumption. It is also a central stimulant and can cause agitation, thus increasing the difficulties of management.

Indications for ventilatory support

The indications for mechanical assistance vary with the condition causing ventilatory failure. Unfortunately, the decision to initiate more active treatment must often be taken on the basis of clinical impression, which is highly subjective. There are some useful guidelines which may be refined when more objective measurements (of respiratory muscle fatigue, for example) become available. The indications for starting support depend not only on the nature of the disease process but also on the presence of other complications and the patient's age and psychological state. The medical history is of particular importance in patients with chronic obstructive airways disease or asthma, and the nature of the surgery and likely surgical complications often affect the decision to provide respiratory support in patients after operation. Serial spirometry and blood gas measurements can be very helpful in assessing the evolution of the disease process, and the non-respiratory component of acid-base balance may provide valuable information concerning the chronicity of CO_2 retention.

The results of a single blood gas measurement should be viewed with caution, not only because of the possibility of sampling, storage, or analytical errors but also because the result may be affected by breath holding or hyperventilation if the sample has been obtained by inexperienced staff. Whenever possible the patient should be observed carefully in the intensive care unit before treatment is started—the response to a period of effective conservative treatment may provide a useful guide to the patient's likely response to more active measures.

Ventilatory failure in patients with normal lungs

Drug overdose. Barbiturate overdose, which used to be the most common condition requiring treatment, has now been superceded by poisoning by the benzodiazepines, tricyclic antidepressants, and opioid and hallucinogenic drugs. Overdose with opioid drugs can usually be managed by giving oxygen, routine care of the unconscious patient, and giving specific antagonists. However, in gross overdose mechanical support may be required to cover a period of prolonged apnoea. Mechanical ventilation may also be required for the treatment of the pulmonary oedema, which is not infrequently observed in patients with heroin overdose.

170

Head injury or other intracranial disease. Patients with intracranial disease such as encephalitis often develop respiratory depression with respiratory irregularities or episodes of central apnoea during sleep. Those with a diminished level of consciousness secondary to intracranial disease will often require endotracheal intubation to prevent the aspiration of pharyngeal contents. Mechanical assistance may be required in patients with increased intracracranial pressure due to head injury or intracranial surgery to ensure that the cerebrospinal fluid pressure is not increased by an increase in arterial PCO_2; in some centres, hyperventilation will be induced in an attempt to lower cerebrospinal fluid pressure. The decision to ventilate is thus based on the results of blood gas analysis and on the intracerebral condition. In general, those with a Glasgow coma score of 8 or less will require ventilatory support.

Paralytic diseases. Patients with respiratory muscle weakness may not seem breathless when resting in bed and may have a normal PCO_2 when the vital capacity has been reduced to 15–20% of normal. This level of disability is associated with considerable reduction in the effectiveness of the cough mechanism, and this often leads to the development of chest infections which may compromise subsequent treatment. Regular measurements of vital capacity are therefore an essential guide to treatment in patients developing respiratory muscle weakness.

If a portable spirometer is not available, useful clinical information can be obtained by asking the patient to take a deep breath and then to breathe out slowly while counting at a rate of about one count per second. By comparing the number of counts produced by the patient with those resulting from a similar manoeuvre performed by the clinician, a rough indication of vital capacity can be obtained. Since a vital capacity of about one quarter of normal (that is, about 20 ml/kg) is required to maintain an efficient cough mechanism, it is usual to start mechanical ventilation when the vital capacity approaches this level. When charts of normal vital capacity values are not available it is useful to remember that the vital capacity is approximately the same as the blood volume (80 ml/kg).

Blood gas measurements are of little value in predicting the need for ventilatory support in patients with paralytic diseases since the PCO_2 often remains normal until the vital capacity falls to very low levels. Indeed, PCO_2 values are usually below normal during the onset of paralysis, probably because patients tend to hyperventilate from anxiety as they feel the paralysis developing. In the later stages, when the tidal volume becomes inadequate to eliminate the CO_2 production, there is usually a rapid rise in PCO_2.

Respiratory weakness in patients with myasthenia gravis is often complicated by profuse secretions resulting from the drug therapy. Since respiratory support is usually required only to cover an acute episode, which can usually be handled with a tracheal tube, and since the presence of secretions increases

Indications for ventilatory support

Respiratory centre depression
 Apnoea, sleep apnoea
 $PaCO_2 > 7-8$ kPa

Increased intracranial pressure
 After trauma, cardiac arrest, neurosurgery
 Glasgow coma score < 8

Cervical cord damage above C4

Paralytic diseases
 Vital capacity $<20-30$ ml/kg (higher if secretions excessive)

Chest wall trauma
 Flail segment
 Severe contusion
 Failure to clear secretions

Acute lung disease
 Respiratory distress
 $PaCO_2 > 7-8$ kPa, $PaO_2 < 8$ kPa on 50% oxygen

Acute exacerbation of chronic lung disease
 Respiratory distress
 Failure to cough
 Decreasing level of consciousness
 Increasing $PaCO_2$ on controlled oxygen therapy

Asthma
 Exhaustion
 $PaCO_2 > 8-9$ kPa, $PaO_2 < 8$ kPa on 50% oxygen

Adult respiratory distress syndrome, pulmonary oedema
 Respiratory distress
 Failure to respond to diuretic and cardiac drugs
 $PaCO_2 > 7-8$ kPa, $PaO_2 < 8$ kPa on 50% oxygen and CPAP

the risk of chest complications, mechanical assistance may be considered at an earlier stage than in patients developing poliomyelitis or polyneuritis. Most units treating myasthenic patients now have facilities for plasmaphere-sis, and this has greatly reduced the need for emergency ventilation.

Tetanus. Patients with tetanus are initially treated by sedation, but if the spasms are uncontrolled they will require total paralysis with a neuromus-cular blocking agent and mechanical ventilation. The disease is usually most severe when the incubation time is short (less than one week from the time of wounding to the onset of the first symptom) and the period of onset (from the first symptom to the first spasm) is less than three days. However, death may occur during the first spasm. In severe cases treatment may need to be continued for three to four weeks.

Respiratory failure in patients with lung disease

Cardiogenic pulmonary oedema. Patients with pulmonary oedema due to acute overload of the circulation or to acute left ventricular failure develop cyanosis, dyspnoea, and wheezing, with the expectoration of bloodstained fluid. There is severe hypoxaemia with a low PCO_2 in the early stages. As the work of breathing increases with the reduction in lung compliance and increase in airway resistance, arterial PCO_2 rises. If the arterial PO_2 remains low after treatment with oxygen and the appropriate diuretics and cardiac drugs, mask CPAP should be initiated. Mechanical ventilation with PEEP should be considered if the arterial PO_2 remains below 8 kPa (60 mm Hg) when the patient is breathing approximately 50% oxygen through the CPAP system. Respiratory fatigue and an increase in PCO_2 above 7–8 kPa are definite indications for mechanical ventilatory support.

ARDS. The characteristic feature of the early stages of ARDS is a low pressure oedema due to increased permeability of the alveolar capillary membrane. There is evidence that this may develop within a few hours of the initial insult, whether this be aspiration of gastric contents, sepsis, massive blood transfusion, viral pneumonia, or some other cause. The pattern of changes is similar to that seen in cardiogenic oedema, and similar indications for CPAP and mechanical assistance apply. In many patients with the syndrome there is very severe hypoxaemia and, later, multiorgan failure. This is associated with a high mortality.

Pneumonia. The predominant blood gas change in pneumonia is hypoxaemia. This is due to an increase in intrapulmonary shunt from the consolidated areas of lung. Reflex stimuli from the lung and peripheral chemoreflex stimuli may cause arterial PCO_2 to be low throughout the acute stage of the disease, so an increase in PCO_2 is a definite indication for mechanical assistance. In patients with widespread disease the arterial PO_2 may be reduced to levels that compromise oxygen delivery to the tissues. Under such circumstances it may be necessary to institute mechanical ventilation in order to be able to apply the appropriate degree of PEEP.

Asthma. In an acute attack of asthma the smaller airways become congested, narrowed, and blocked with mucus plugs. This results in a large increase in airways resistance and work of breathing, overdistension of the lungs, gross ventilation-perfusion inequalities, and an increase in intrapulmonary shunt. A reduction in arterial PO_2 occurs early in the attack, and PO_2 may remain low even when high concentrations of oxygen are given. Since

173

the use of mechanical ventilation often results in a decrease in cardiac output, further lung distension, and barotrauma, its use should be limited to the few patients who fail to maintain adequate alveolar ventilation or who develop a reduced level of consciousness because of severe hypoxaemia.

The appropriate moment for intervention is difficult to assess because severe cases develop marked respiratory distress and exhaustion, and when ventilatory failure occurs it does so rapidly.[12] Frequent monitoring of the PCO_2 is therefore required, and treatment should be instituted when PCO_2 shows a rapid upward trend. In some centres a regimen of "permissive hypercapnia" is used, the arterial PCO_2 being allowed to rise to levels of 7–8 kPa (50–60 mm Hg) or more before intervention is considered. Peak and mean airway pressures may be minimised by maintaining these levels throughout the acute phase of the illness.

Acute-on-chronic chest disease. Most patients with acute exacerbations of chronic chest disease can be managed with antibiotic and bronchodilator drugs, controlled oxygen therapy, and vigorous physiotherapy. In some units respiratory stimulants are given as well. In other units non-invasive mechanical support is provided by face mask or nasal mask.[11] This support is particularly useful during sleep and may prevent a further increase in PCO_2 at this time. Most of these patients have a chronically increased PCO_2, so this in itself is not an indication for more active treatment.

Conservative treatment is considered to have failed when the patient's level of consciousness decreases to such an extent that the secretions cannot be cleared by coughing. This usually occurs when the arterial PCO_2 exceeds 10 kPa (80 mm Hg). It is important to ascertain that the patient has a reasonable level of lung function between attacks before initiating intubation and mechanical assistance. Treatment not only causes patients with grossly impaired chronic lung function a great deal of unnecessary discomfort but is also likely to result in an inability to wean the patient from the ventilator.[13,14]

Postoperative pulmonary complications. It is now known that about 95% of patients undergoing major abdominal surgery in the supine position develop a compression collapse in the dependent regions of the lungs and that these changes persist for several days after operation. The early changes are usually not visible on the standard posteroanterior chest radiograph because they occur in the areas of lung in close proximity to the paracolic gutters and thus do not cause localised opacities when viewed from the front. However, basal collapse is often apparent on the postoperative radiograph when the patient sits up.

The cause of the collapse is still not known, but it is most likely to occur in patients who undergo upper abdominal surgery. A history of smoking, obesity, intra-abdominal distension, and sepsis are factors that increase the frequency and severity of the lung changes, which usually peak on the first and second postoperative days but may persist for 5–10 days.

Recent studies using continuous pulse oximetry recording have shown that there are frequently additional dips in arterial saturation during sleep. These are due to episodes of central depression and upper airway obstruction associated with the use of postoperative analgesic drugs.[2] In the absence of oxygen therapy they may result in dips in saturation to levels of 60–70%.

Patients with such complications require continuous oxygen therapy (especially at night) for several days after operation, together with vigorous physiotherapy and possibly bronchodilators and antibiotics. Bronchoscopy, or manual hyperventilation and suction though an endotracheal tube, may be required to help re-expand collapsed areas of lung. The indications for mechanical assistance are a decreasing level of consciousness, an inability to cough, exhaustion, and a rising PCO_2 and, occasionally, a persistent, severe degree of hypoxaemia which requires treatment with PEEP.

Chest trauma. Blunt trauma to the chest wall may result in fractured ribs, diaphragmatic rupture, damage to the major vessels or heart, haemothorax or pneumothorax, bronchopleural fistula, and lung contusion. There may also be injuries to the head and other parts of the body. Tracheal intubation may be required to secure an airway and to prevent the aspiration of blood, gastric contents, and secretions, but positive pressure should not be applied to the airway until the extent of the damage has been ascertained and preparations made for chest drainage. At one time a floating area of chest wall was considered to be an indication for mechanical ventilation with low level PEEP, but it is now recognised that many patients with this complication can be treated with conservative measures provided that good pain relief is obtained by the use of intravenous opiates, patient controlled analgesia, intercostal blocks, or epidural blocks with local analgesics or opioid drugs.[15,16]

Conclusions

The indications for mechanical assistance in all these forms of respiratory failure depend on many factors. The age and general condition of the patient are important, but even more important is the patient's psychological approach to treatment. Local environmental factors may influence the incidence of chronic chest disease or other disease, and the availability of trained nursing and medical staff and equipment may ultimately dictate the pattern of treatment. Nevertheless, a rational decision can be taken only if the physician has a firm grasp of the basic physiology and of the clinical course of the diseases being treated. Although improved methods of clinical measurement may provide more information on which to base our decisions, there is a great need for more careful documentation of the indications for mechanical assistance in each patient, so that this data can be correlated with short term and long term survival.

1 Kelly BJ, Luce JM. The diagnosis and management of neuromuscular diseases causing respiratory failure. *Chest* 1991;**99**:1485–94.
2 Reeder MK, Goldman MD, Loh L, Muir AD, Foëx P, Casey KR, *et al.* Postoperative hypoxaemia after major abdominal vascular surgery. *Br J Anaesth* 1992;**68**:23–6.
3 Goldman MD. Neuromuscular respiratory failure. *Care of the Critically Ill* 1989;**5**: 131–3.
4 Howard RS, Wiles CM, Loh L. Respiratory complications and their management in motor neurone disease. *Brain* 1989;**112**:1155–70.
5 Lassen HCA. A preliminary report on the 1952 epidemic of poliomyelitis in Copenhagen with special reference to the treatment of acute respiratory insufficiency. *Lancet* 1953;i: 37–41.
6 Gracey DR, McMichan JC, Divertie MB, Howard FM. Respiratory failure in Guillain–Barré syndrome: a six year experience. *Mayo Clin Proc* 1982;**57**:742–6.
7 Roelofs RI. Critical illness polyneuropathy. *Chest* 1991;**99**:5–6.
8 Smith CL, Hunter JM, Jones RS. Vecuronium infusions in patients in renal failure in an ICU. *Anaesthesia* 1987;**42**:387–93.
9 Margolis BD, Khachikian D, Friedman Y, Garrard C. Prolonged reversible quadriparesis in mechanically ventilated patients who received long-term infusions of vecuronium. *Chest* 1991;**100**:877–8.
10 Goldstone J, Moxham J. Weaning from mechanical ventilation. In: Moxham J, Goldstone J, eds. *Assisted Ventilation*. London: BMJ Publications, 1994:57–79.
11 Brochard L, Isabey D, Piquet J, Amaro P, Mancebo J, Messadi AA, *et al.* Reversal of acute exacerbations of chronic obstructive lung disease by inspiratory assistance with a face mask. *N Engl J Med* 1990;**323**:1523–30.
12 Higgins B, Greening AP, Crompton GL. Assisted ventilation in acute severe asthma. *Thorax* 1986;**41**:464–7.
13 Muir JF, Levi-Valenci P. When should patients with COPD be ventilated? *Eur J Resp Dis* 1987;**70**:135–9.
14 Menzies R, Gibbons W, Goldberg P. Determinants of weaning and survival among patients with severe COPD who require mechanical ventilation for acute respiratory failure. *Chest* 1990;**95**:398–405.
15 Richardson JD, Adams I, Flint LM. Selective management of flail chest and pulmonary contusion. *Ann Sug* 1982;**196**:481-7.
16 Mackenzie RC, Shackford SR, Hoyt DB, Karagianes TG. Continuous epidural fentanyl analgesia: ventilatory function improvement with routine use in the treatment of blunt chest injury. *J Trauma* 1987;**27**:1207-12.

8 Selection and care of artificial airways

In conscious patients a connection between the gas source and lungs can be secured by a face mask, nasal mask, or mouthpiece, or by nasal prongs. These are used with non-invasive methods of respiratory support and are described in chapter 10.

In unconscious patients or in those requiring ventilatory assistance for more prolonged periods the choice of airway lies between a pharyngeal airway, laryngeal mask airway, nasal or oral intubation, or tracheostomy (box).

The oral airway

The maintenance of a patent airway is one of the major problems in the care of the unconscious patient. All non-intubated unconscious patients should be nursed on their side unless there is some contraindication (for

---

Choice of airway

Pharyngeal airway, laryngeal mask
   For emergency situation

Tracheal intubation
- Oral
   Emergency and short term
   In patients in whom nasal route is contraindicated
- Nasal
   Neonates
   Children and adults where possible
   For treatment up to 7-10 days

Tracheostomy
   For patients with severe maxillofacial injuries
   When there is laryngeal damage
   When support is needed for more than one week
   When CPAP is required for chest trauma

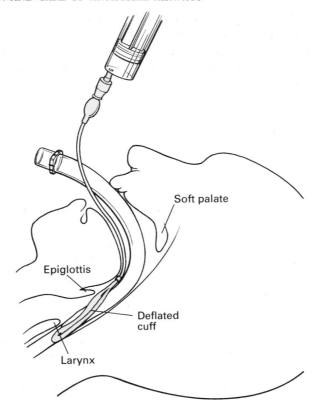

Fig 8.1 Laryngeal mask airway. Mask is inserted into pharynx with its concavity facing anteriorly to form airtight seal around epiglottis and larynx.

example, a possible cervical spine injury). In the lateral position the tongue tends to fall sideways and the risk of aspiration is reduced. The risk of aspiration can be reduced further by the head down position. In many patients obstruction of the airway due to the tongue falling back onto the posterior pharyngeal wall can be prevented by simple extension of the head. If this manoeuvre does not secure a clear airway it will be necessary to push the jaw forward by pressure on the posterior ramus of the mandible. However, pressure on the mandible tends to close the mouth, and this may increase airway obstruction if the patient has blocked nasal passages. Under these circumstances it may be necessary to insert a pharyngeal airway to maintain an air passage through the mouth.

The laryngeal mask airway (fig 8.1) has revolutionised anaesthetic practice: it can be inserted without using a laryngoscope, and the inflatable cuff provides a relatively airtight seal within the pharynx. However, some skill is required to ensure that it is correctly positioned, and it can be tolerated only by an unconscious or anaesthetised patient. Furthermore, air leaks tend to occur if airway pressures exceed 15–20 cm H_2O, and the aspiration of oral secretions or gastric contents is always a possibility.[1] Although the device may prove lifesaving in patients who are difficult to intubate, it is unlikely to displace tracheal intubation in intensive care practice.

Tracheal intubation

Choice of route

The oral route is preferred for an emergency intubation since the tracheal tube can be passed quickly and tracheobronchial toilet can be performed easily. The oral route is less suitable for prolonged use as the presence of the tube often causes discomfort, nausea, vomiting, or coughing; fixation can prove difficult; and the tube may be occluded by biting or by kinking as it passes round the base of the tongue. A nasal tube is more secure and causes the patient less discomfort, but it is longer than an oral tube, and in adults the nasal passages are often narrowed by the turbinates or by a deviated septum. Both these factors increase tube resistance and hinder the aspiration of secretions. Another problem is that infection of the sinuses occurs in a proportion of patients, particularly if the patient has received steroids[2]; also, ulceration of the nasal mucous membrane is not infrequent.

In neonates and children up to 2 years the nasal passages tend to have a larger cross-sectional area than the cricoid ring, so that narrowing of the tube within the nose is uncommon. The baby's skin is delicate, the skull is easily deformed, and fixation of an oral tube is difficult. Furthermore, the trachea bifurcates at T2 in the neonate (as opposed to T4 in the adult) so there is a high risk of endobronchial intubation if the tube is not firmly anchored. In neonates and children a tube without a cuff is used and the tube size is adjusted to ensure that there is a slight leak around the tube during inflation. This ensures that the tube does not press on the cricoid cartilage and cause subglottic oedema and, later, stenosis.[3]

Because of these considerations most units use a nasal tube for neonates and children.[4] An oral tube is used in adults if the period of ventilation is likely to be measured in hours rather than days, but for longer periods a nasal tube is preferred, providing the anatomy of the nasal passage permits a tube of adequate diameter to be tolerated.

Choice of tube

In neonates and infants it is common to use the pressure generation mode, which compensates for the small leak that occurs when a loosely fitting

179

uncuffed tube is used, but in adults it is usual to insert a cuffed tube. The early cuffed tubes were made of red rubber, which irritated tissues. Their small cuffs required a high pressure for inflation. The inflated cuff assumed a spherical shape and so tended to produce an area of high pressure on the mucosa, with resulting ulceration. A variation in cuff wall thickness often made the cuff inflate unevenly, so causing the tip of the tube to press on the trachea and create another area of ulceration. Although most of the force generated by the high intracuff pressure was exerted against the elasticity of the rubber, and it was possible to ensure that the mucosa was not unduly compressed by inflating the cuff very carefully, it was not possible to determine what pressure was being exerted on the mucosa.

Capillary blood flow ceases when a pressure greater than 25–30 cm H_2O is applied to the mucosa,[5] while a minimum pressure of approximately 25 cm H_2O is required to prevent the aspiration of secretions past the cuff.[6] The only practicable way of achieving this is to ensure that the pressure difference across the wall of the inflated cuff is small, so that the intracuff pressure may be used as a measure of the pressure applied to the mucosa. The earliest designs of low pressure cuffs had a large volume and cylindrical shape. Since the diameter of the cuff exceeded that of the trachea, the cuff wall was not stretched when fully inflated. These cuffs were difficult to pass through the larynx, and the excess material in the cuff formed creases which resulted in a poor seal with the trachea. With improved technology, manufacturers can produce cuffs with a smaller volume but a high compliance, so that intracuff pressure may still be used as a measure of the pressure applied to the tracheal mucosa.

At first sight, it is surprising that an intracuff pressure of 25–30 cm H_2O can maintain an airtight seal when the airway pressure may peak at 50–60 cm H_2O. The explanation (fig 8.2) is that when the tracheal pressure exceeds cuff pressure the lower part of the cuff is compressed so that cuff pressure increases in proportion to airway pressure.[7] The cyclical increase in pressure probably decreases capillary blood flow during part of the respiratory cycle, but it is believed that this is less damaging than the continuous pressure exerted by a high pressure cuff.

Several special tubes may be utilised in the operating room and so may be present in patients who are transferred to the intensive care unit. Latex or plastic armoured tubes have a wire or plastic spiral incorporated in the wall to prevent kinking when the patient's head is placed in an abnormal position. They are often used during head and neck surgery. Oxford tubes were also designed to minimise obstruction due to kinking and have a right angled bend instead of a curve. This shape probably also minimises pressure on the posterior part of the vocal cords, an area that is particularly prone to damage from the backward pressure exerted by conventional curved tubes. The disadvantage of the Oxford tube is that a stylet is required to facilitate insertion, and it is difficult to alter the position of the tip of the tube in the

Types of tracheal tube

Plastic noncuffed
  Used in neonates and infants

Plastic cuffed
  High pressure cuffs damage tracheal mucosa
  With low pressure cuffs intracuff pressure can be used as a measure of
  pressure applied to tracheal mucosa

Latex or plastic armoured tubes
  Prevent kinking when head is in abnormal position

Oxford tubes
  Right angled bend minimises risk of kinking and decreases pressure on
  posterior part of vocal cords

Special tubes
  For measurement of tracheal pressure
  For high frequency jet ventilation

Single and double lumen endobronchial tubes
  For thoracic surgery and differential lung ventilation

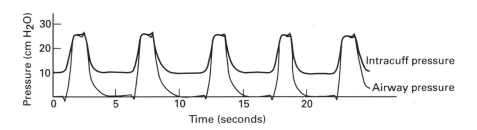

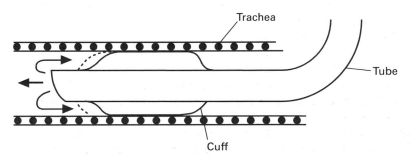

Fig 8.2 (top) Variations in cuff pressure with airway pressure (after Crawley and Cross[7])
(bottom). Cuff pressure increases because the airway pressure deforms the cuff from its
original shape (dotted line).

181

trachea because the distance between the right angled bend and tube tip is fixed in relation to tube size.

A special tube is used for high frequency jet ventilation. This usually consists of a standard cuffed tracheal tube with the narrow bore jet tube and a pressure measurement tube incorporated in the wall. The jet tube discharges into the main tube about 10 cm from its outer end and the pressure tube senses the airway pressure at the patient's end of the tracheal tube. Another recent introduction is a tracheal tube with a single pressure sensing tube incorporated in the wall: this enables lower airway pressure to be measured. Pressure measurement at this position reduces the delay between the initiation of inspiration and the ventilator response when patient triggering is used, and inspiratory pressure support can be set at a level that compensates for the work of breathing generated by the resistance of the breathing system and tracheal tube (chapter 6).

Various single and double lumen endobronchial tubes are used during thoracic surgery. Double lumen endobronchial tubes are also used during differential lung ventilation and have been described in chapter 4.

Complications

The common complications of intubation are damage to the lips or teeth, intubation of the oesophagus, and endobronchial intubation. None of the clinical signs purporting to confirm successful tracheal intubation (chest movements, breath sounds over the lung fields, recoil of the reservoir bag) has proved to be completely reliable, and it is now agreed that the only certain way of checking that the tube is in the trachea is to establish that an end tidal plateau of CO_2 can be identified by the use of a rapid gas analyser over several breaths. (CO_2 is often present in gas from the stomach, but the concentration falls rapidly with successive breaths.) Other devices such as the commercially available colorimetric detectors or the syringe detector device[8] may be substituted in an emergency.

Endobronchial intubation is surprisingly common, probably because of a conscious attempt to prevent accidental extubation by ensuring that the tube is not too short. It is especially common in elderly patients (who often have a small mandible due to bone resorption) and in patients with short necks. The tube usually enters the right main bronchus, because this tends to diverge from the axis of the trachea at a smaller angle than the left, and the bevel of the tube faces the left. If the tip of the tube lies more than 1–2 cm below the carina, the end opening may be occluded by the medial wall of the right main bronchus. This often creates a valvular effect, inspired gas passing freely into the bronchus, but expiration being impeded by the apposition of the tube opening to the bronchial mucosa. This occurrence can often be detected by hearing loud rhonchi during expiration together with hyperinflation of the right lung. Endobronchial intubation leads to arterial desaturation, but this may take one or two minutes to develop if the patient has been breathing high concentrations of oxygen. The arterial saturation should therefore be measured continuously whenever possible. It should be routine practice after every intubation to auscultate both lung fields (especially over the upper lobes in the axillae), and wherever possible the position of the tube should be checked by radiography.[9]

Laryngeal damage. All patients who have been intubated suffer some degree of laryngeal damage. If the period of intubation has been short the damage may be limited to a mild inflammation of the vocal cords, with subsequent slight hoarseness. In neonates and young children subglottic oedema may develop, particularly if the tube has been too large and has pressed on the mucosa in the region of the cricoid cartilage. The oedema may develop immediately after extubation or over the next 24 hours.

With an increased duration of intubation more severe laryngeal lesions are seen. The cords are inflamed and there may be ulceration, particularly on the

---

Complications of tracheal intubation[10–13]

During use
    Damage to lips and teeth
    Intubation of oesophagus
        Verify position by end tidal PCO_2
    Accidental extubation
    Endobronchial intubation
        Common in neonates, elderly patients, and those with short necks
        Check length before insertion
        Check position by:
            Chest movements
            Auscultation over upper and lower lobes of both lungs
            Radiography
            Compliance measurement
            Oxygen saturation
    Blockage of end opening
        By medial wall of right main bronchus
        By herniation of cuff over end of tube
    Narrowing of tube by kinking or external compression
    Blockage by blood clot, inspissated secretions, or foreign body
    Aspiration of pharyngeal contents or gas leak past deflated cuff

Long term
    Chest infection
    Laryngeal damage
    Tracheal damage
        From pressure of cuff or tip of tube
        From use of suction catheter with end hole only

posterior third where maximum pressure is exerted due to the reversal of the natural curvature of the tube as it enters the larynx. These ulcers may subsequently give rise to papillomata, abnormalities of cord movement, and even vocal cord paralysis.[11,12] Ulceration of the skin and pharyngeal and nasal mucosa also occurs, particularly if the patient is hypotensive for more than a short period.

Extubation

Extubation should be considered when the patient has been satisfactorily weaned from respiratory support and when secretions are unlikely to create a problem. Ideally, extubation should be performed in the earlier part of the day so that complications can be detected and treated under optimum conditions. Extubation should be peformed after tracheobronchial toilet has been carried out and the alveolar oxygen concentration has been increased to a maximum by breathing oxygen. Oxygen therapy should then be continued until the patient seems to be breathing normally and the arterial saturation is satisfactory. Close observation of the patient is necessary for the next 12–24 hours, for laryngeal function is usually impaired by a period of intubation of more than a few hours. Post-extubation stridor is most common in neonates and children and should be treated with oxygen, high humidity, and steroids. If the stridor leads to respiratory distress it may be necessary to reintubate the trachea for a further 24 hours and to give steroids before attempting extubation again.

Tracheostomy

Indications

There are four main indications for performing a tracheostomy (box).

Indications for tracheostromy

- To bypass an upper respiratory tract obstruction
- To prevent aspiration from pharynx in patients with chronic bulbar palsy
- To facilitate aspiration of secretions from trachea
- To provide an airway for provision of respiratory support
- To reduce dead space (rare)

A tracheostomy may also be of value in reducing dead space in patients with respiratory failure due to chronic obstructive airways disease. However, the reduction in dead space is small (< 70 ml) and this constitutes a relatively small proportion of the greatly enlarged physiological dead space which is usually present. Furthermore, such patients tend to decrease their ventilation after tracheostomy, so that the PCO_2 returns to the pre-existing level after the operation. One of the few situations in which the reduction in dead space may prove valuable is to tide the patient over a short period of increased airway obstruction. For example, patients with a lower respiratory tract obstruction due to a carcinoma may develop increased obstruction when they undergo radiotherapy. Under these circumstances a preliminary tracheostomy may alleviate much distress.

Tracheostomy versus tracheal intubation

The main advantage of tracheal intubation over tracheostomy is that the complications associated with an open wound are avoided. In one prospective study tracheostomy was associated with a 36% rate of moderate to severe stomal haemorrhage and a 36% incidence of stomal infection,[12] but in another study in which a limited number of surgeons performed the operation, the incidence of major morbidity was less than 2%.[13] Tracheal intubation has many disadvantages: it is uncomfortable for the patient; tube fixation is difficult; there is a high incidence of sinusitis in patients with nasal intubations[2]; and laryngeal complications are not infrequent.[11] It is generally believed that the incidence of laryngeal complications increases with the duration of intubation, but there is little evidence to support this contention,[14] and laryngeal stenosis, glottic incompetence, vocal cord paralysis, voice abnormalities, and dysphagia have been recorded after intubation for 1–3 days.[15,16] Although it has been suggested that chest infection is more common after tracheostomy than intubation, many of the studies are biased by the inclusion of more seriously ill patients in the tracheostomy group.[14]

In view of the conflicting evidence, one must take a pragmatic approach in deciding when to perform a tracheostomy. The first consideration is the nature of the disease process. For example, there is no point in delaying the tracheostomy in a patient with severe tetanus or the Guillain-Barré syndrome, since treatment will usually be required for a period of several weeks. Patients with a severe chest injury treated by continuous positive pressure breathing often find a tracheostomy more comfortable than a tracheal tube and usually require less sedation, so early tracheostomy is again advised. An early tracheostomy is also a wise precaution in patients with severe maxillofacial injuries and in those who are disorientated by head injury. In other patients it is usually best to start treatment with a tracheal tube and to consider tracheostomy after 7–10 days of treatment, when the prognosis will usually be more clearly defined.

185

Tracheostomy techniques

Emergency
  Cricothyroidotomy or tracheostomy

Mini-tracheostomy
  Used in patients who require chronic oxygen therapy or repeated aspiration
  of secretions

Percutaneous
  Can be performed in intensive care unit

Surgical operation
  Under local anaesthesia
  Under general anaesthesia

Tracheostomy techniques

Emergency. In an emergency oxygen can be supplied to the trachea using a 14 or 12 gauge needle or cannula (internal diameter 2.5 or 3.5 mm) inserted through the cricothyroid membrane.[17] The cannula can be connected to a high pressure gas source (such as that used to drive a Sanders injector or high frequency jet ventilator) and the lungs ventilated by admitting pulses of gas into the trachea. Tidal volume is controlled by close observation of chest movement. Since the only expiratory pathway is through the larynx, it is vital to ensure that there is a free passage for exhaled gases. An alternative is to perform a cricothyroidotomy with one of the commercially available devices.

Mini-tracheostomy. This technique is used when frequent tracheal suction or the administration of oxygen is needed in patients with excessive secretions. A 4 mm internal diameter plastic cannula is inserted through the cricothyroid membrane under local anaesthesia by using either surgical incision of the membrane[18] or placement with a Seldinger wire guide.[19] The procedure must be carried out with care, for a number of complications have been reported. The small internal diameter of the tube limits the size of suction catheter that may be passed: the external diameter of the catheter should be no more than half the internal diameter of the tube to prevent collapse of the lungs when suction is applied. The small diameter also increases the risk of tube blockage if secretions are viscous. In skilled hands mini-tracheostomy may be a useful alternative to a surgical tracheostomy.[20]

Percutaneous tracheostomy. In recent years various techniques of percutaneous tracheostomy have been introduced. In all these techniques the pretracheal tissues are incised under local anaesthesia and a Seldinger guide wire is inserted into the trachea, usually below the first or second tracheal rings.[21] The trachea is dilated with special forceps or with conical dilators that are slipped over the guide wire, and a standard tracheostomy tube is inserted over the largest dilator. The main advantage of this technique is that the operation can be performed in the intensive care unit. It is also claimed that the minimal dissection of the pretracheal tissues decreases the incidence of complications.[22] However, it is extremely difficult to design a trial that would provide a valid comparison between the standard and percutaneous routes because of the many variables that affect the outcome.[23]

Surgical operation. The operation should ideally be performed under general anaesthesia in the operating theatre. In patients with upper respiratory tract obstruction it is wise to intubate the trachea under a topical anaesthetic to minimise the risk of complete airway obstruction. When this is difficult, inhalation anaesthesia with spontaneous ventilation may be used. In most other cases the trachea can be intubated under an intravenous anaesthetic and muscle relaxant and anaesthesia maintained with a light inhalational anaesthetic. Although it is theoretically safer to maintain spontaneous respiration throughout the operation, controlled ventilation is usually preferred for it enables the respiratory failure to be corrected immediately and provides superior operating conditions. However, when the patient has developed compensatory non-respiratory acid-base changes for a high PCO_2, it is important not to reduce PCO_2 too quickly because this may reduce cerebral blood flow and cause cerebral damage.

To minimise bleeding and provide optimal surgical access a head up tilt should be used. The head should be extended at the atlanto-occipital joint and the cervical vertebrae flexed (the normal position for tracheal intubation). A transverse skin incision is used, the thyroid isthmus divided (to reduce the risk of secondary haemorrhage), and the tracheostomy inserted at the level of the second to the fourth tracheal rings. When the surgeon has tested the tracheostomy tube cuff and is ready to insert the tube, the table is tilted 20° head down, the tracheal tube cuff is deflated, and the tube withdrawn so that its tip is just above the tracheostomy opening. The tracheostomy tube is then inserted and the cuff is inflated and its position checked by auscultating in both axillae while manual ventilation is performed. The tip of the tracheal tube should be left within the larynx until the patient has been connected to the ventilator in the intensive care unit so that it can easily be pushed down into the trachea should the tracheostomy tube become displaced during transport. A spare tracheostomy tube, with suitable equipment for replacing it, should accompany the patient at all times.

Complications of tracheostomy

Some of the common complications of tracheostomy are shown in figure 8.3.[12,13] Disconnection is a major hazard, but the risk can be minimised by

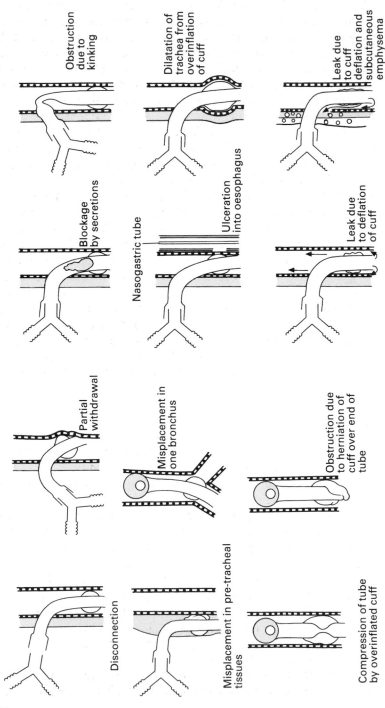

Fig 8.3 Some complications of tracheostomy.

using a clip to secure the connection between tube and ventilator and by using a disconnect alarm. The tube can be misplaced into the pretracheal tissues when it is changed and also if the tube is partially dragged out of the trachea by the weight of the ventilator tubes and then replaced by an inexperieced attendant. This complication is much more likely if the wound is covered by surgical dressings that conceal the position of the tube. Tubes may be blocked by blood clots, dried secretions, overinflation of the cuff, or endobronchial intubation. Optimal humidification is required at all times, but aliquots of saline may need to be injected into the trachea at frequent intervals if secretions thicken or bleeding from the lung occurs. Tracheal lesions may result from improper suction techniques, and infection, both in the wound and in the lungs, is an ever present problem.

The use of implant-tested plastics and low pressure cuffs has reduced the incidence of tracheal ulceration at the site of the cuff, but ulceration may also occur at the site of the tracheostomy opening and at the level of the tip of the tube. Ulceration may lead to bleeding and the erosion of the tracheal cartilages and neighbouring structures. Fatal haemorrhages from the innominate artery and tracheo-oesophageal fistulae have been recorded. Ulceration may also progress to tracheal stenosis, which may not become apparent until months after treatment. Surprisingly, patients do not usually present for treatment of the stenosis until its diameter approaches 15–20% of the diameter of the trachea. Mild degrees of stenosis may respond to dilation but more severe stenoses will require surgical resection. In patients with a chronic tracheostomy gradual dilation of the trachea at the site of the cuff may occur.

Tracheostomy care

The wound should be sealed with a plastic dressing at operation and this should not be disturbed unless obvious infection develops. Unless an emergency occurs, the tracheostomy tube should not be changed until a well defined track has formed. This takes four to five days. When rubber tracheostomy tubes with high pressure cuffs were in use it was customary to deflate the cuff for a few minutes every four hours (to try and prevent mucosal damage) and to change the tube every few days, but now the only reason for changing a tube is blockage or cuff failure.

If the tube has to be changed, full emergency precautions should be taken. There should be a selection of tracheal tubes, appropriate anaesthetic agents, apparatus for manually inflating the lungs and equipment for emergency oral intubation, should it prove impossible to reinsert the tracheostomy tube. Tracheal dilators, a range of tracheostomy tubes and gum elastic bougies, and suction apparatus should be available.

The trachea should be cleared of secretions by tracheobronchial toilet and a high concentration of oxygen given for several minutes before the procedure.

189

> ## Types of tracheostomy tube
>
> Metal
> > Semicircular or "lobster tail"
> > With removable inner tube
> > With valved inner tube for speech
>
> Plastic
> > With integral cuff
> > With removable inner tube and hole in outer tube for weaning

A bougie with a diameter about half that of the internal diameter of the tube should then be inserted into the trachea through the old tracheostomy tube, to act as a guide. The cuff should then be deflated, the old tube slid out of the trachea and the new one slid into place over the bougie. If the wound is small it may be necessary to use tracheal dilators to enlarge the orifice as the tube is slid into place. The cuff is then inflated and the position of the tube checked by auscultation of the lungs, CO_2 analysis, and pulse oximetry.

Tracheostomy tubes

Tracheostomy tubes were originally made of metal and had two concentric tubes, the inner removable for regular cleaning. Some were shaped into a 90° arc of a circle to permit the inner tube to slide within the outer, but tubes with this configuration were not suitable for those with thick pretracheal tissues and frequently became misplaced. The problem was overcome by using a J shaped outer tube with a movable collar which enabled the length of tube within the patient to be matched to the distance of the trachea from the skin (fig 8.4). Such a tube required an inner tube with a flexible tip, the "lobster tail" design.

Metal tubes continued to be used in the early days of intermittent positive pressure ventilation, and an airtight seal was obtained by slipping an inflatable rubber cuff over the outer tube. Unfortunately, this sometimes became detached, with disastrous consequences. By 1953 it had been realised that adequate humidification could prevent the formation of inspissated secretions which caused blockage of the inner tube, so manufacturers started to produce a range of rubber and, later, plastic tubes with an integral cuff. There is now a wide choice of plastic disposable tubes, often fitted with an obturator to facilitate insertion, and most of the larger sizes are available with low pressure cuffs.

Tubes designed to facilitate weaning from a ventilator usually have two concentric tubes, the outer of which has one or more holes situated along the convexity of the curve above the cuff (fig 8.5). The inner tube has no holes

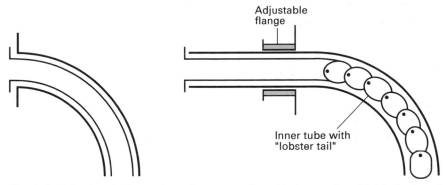

Fig 8.4 (left) Standard metal tracheostomy tube with inner tube. (right) J shaped tracheostomy tube with adjustable collar. The inner tube has a "lobster tail" to enable it to pass through both the straight and curved parts of the outer tube.

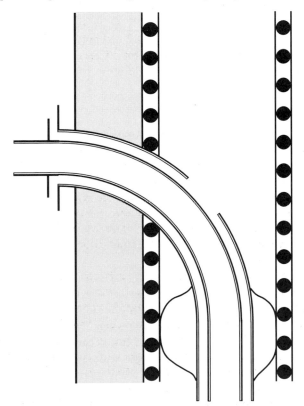

Fig 8.5 Fenestrated speaking tracheostomy tube. When the inner tube is withdrawn and the orifice of the outer tube is blocked, the patient can breathe through larynx and phonate. Alternatively, the inner tube may be replaced by a tube with a one way inlet valve and a hole on the convexity. This permits the patient to breathe in through the tracheostomy and exhale through the larynx.

and is connected to the ventilator. Since it fits tightly into the outer tube it serves as the airway while the patient is being ventilated. When the inner tube is withdrawn the patient can breathe through the larynx as well as the tracheostomy. As confidence is gained the end of the outer tracheostomy tube can be occluded so that the patient can breathe for increasing periods entirely through the larynx. The tube may then be removed.

Patients who require a chronic tracheostomy may use a similar non-cuffed tube and manually occlude the outer end when they wish to speak; they may also use a specially designed talking tube. This consists of an outer tube with a hole on the convexity of the curve. There are two inner tubes: a standard tube, which is used at night, and a speaking tube. The speaking tube has a hole in the convexity that matches the hole in the outer tube, and it has a one way flap valve at its outer end. Air is drawn in through the valve during inspiration but is directed through the holes to the larynx in expiration, thus enabling the patient to speak. Patients on long term ventilation often manage to speak while on a ventilator by partially deflating the cuff. A ventilator, such as the East-Radcliffe, that provides a constant source of pressure during inspiration facilitates speech and also compensates for the leak around the cuff.

General care of the airway

The use of a tracheal or tracheostomy tube causes the inspired and expired gases to bypass the nasopharynx and larynx. Since the nasopharynx filters, warms, and moistens the inspired gas and the larynx is an integral part of the cough mechanism, it is necessary to replace these functions artificially. This is done by providing sterile inspired gas with a high humidity at a temperature of 35–37°C and by using physiotherapy and tracheobronchial suction to transfer the secretions from the airways to the exterior.

Care of the tube

The tube must be securely fixed in position and connected by a flexible connection to the ventilator tubes, which should be supported so that no force is applied to the tube. Oral tubes are usually retained by a tape that passes round the neck, but the patient's comfort can be improved by using a short tape to connect the tube to a 5 cm wide padded rubber strap that encircles the cheeks and neck. When a nasal tube is used in neonates and children security can be increased by fixing the ventilator tubes to each side of the head by means of a head net or a head band made from wide elastic strapping, the area under the tubing being carefully padded.

Contact points between the tube and the skin or mucosa should be examined at frequent intervals and the position changed to avoid pressure necrosis. Regular mouth care is essential when tracheal tubes are used. When a cuffed tube is used the cuff pressure should be maintained at the lowest level that will prevent aspiration and gas leakage from the system (20–25 cm H_2O) and the intracuff pressure should be regularly checked with a pressure gauge.

Prevention of infection

The sterility of the inspired gas should be assured by providing bacterial filters at the input to the ventilator, at the ports connecting the breathing system to the ventilator, or at the patient Y piece. Using filters at the junction between the breathing system and the ventilator obviates the need to sterilise the interior of the ventilator and has the advantage that the weight of the filters is born by the ventilator. However, infection developing in the humidifier may be transmitted to the patient. Filters situated at the patient Y piece eliminate this problem but add to the bulk and weight of the tubes attached to the patient. Condensation is also a problem. Devices combining a filter and a heat and moisture exchanger are now available.[24] These are fitted between the Y piece and the patient and prevent water accumulation in the ventilator tubes. However, the level of inspired humidity obtainable with these devices may not be adequate for patients with increased secretions (see below).

Filters vary in their effectiveness against bacteria, and none of those designed for use in breathing systems are effective against viruses. A filter increases the resistance of the breathing system to a variable degree, and the resistance may be increased by droplets of mucopus deposited on the filter element or by water accumulating within the casing. If filters are incorporated in the breathing system their internal volume will add to the internal compliance of the system. This may result in a decrease in delivered tidal volume and a possible error in tidal volume measurement (see page 66).

The major source of iatrogenic chest infection is probably the passage of a suction catheter for tracheobronchial toilet. Although sterile catheters and a no touch technique may be used, infection is common. The pathogen is often present in the patient's mouth, nose, or other part of the body and could also have been introduced during passage of the tracheal or tracheostomy tube.

Humidification

Principles

There are two measures of humidity: absolute humidity and relative humidity. The absolute humidity is defined as the mass of water contained in unit volume of gas at a given temperature (g/m^3). The relative humidity (or relative saturation) at a given temperature is:

$$\frac{\text{Mass of water in unit volume of gas}}{\text{Mass of water in same volume of gas when fully saturated}} \times 100$$

The mass of water contained in unit volume of fully saturated gas depends on the vapour pressure of the water and therefore increases with temperature (fig 8.6). Air at 37°C contains about 43 g/m^3 (43 mg/l) when it is fully saturated.

Inspired gas is normally warmed and moistened as it passes through the nose and when it reaches the upper trachea has a temperature of 32–36°C and a humidity close to 100%, even when the inspired gas is very cold. The warming and humidification continues as the gas passes down the airways: the gas is fully saturated and at a temperature of 37°C when it reaches the alveoli. As the gas leaves through the nose it is cooled again and gives up about 20% of its water and heat.

Simple calculations show that most of the heat lost from the respiratory tract is used in the vaporisation of water. The specific heat of air is low (0.863 J/l/°C) so the heat required to warm 8 l/min of dry air from, say, 21°C to 37°C is $0.863 \times 8 \times 16 = 110$ J/min. The combined effects of heating and adding water vapour increase the volume so that the total flow is approximately 9 l/min at the lower end of the trachea. The latent heat of vaporisation of water is 2445 J/g so the heat loss from vaporisation is 9 l/min $\times$ 0.043 g/l $\times$ 2445 J/g = 946 J/min. Thus the heat required to warm the air is about one ninth of that required to vaporise the water. In situations where very high minute volumes pass down the trachea (for example, during the use of high frequency jet ventilation or during ventilation of the lungs in patients with a large air leak) the excessive heat loss may result in rapid cooling of the patient. However, if this gas is humidified heat loss is greatly reduced.

The purpose of humidifying the inspired gas is, firstly, to prevent the drying of secretions and, secondly, to maintain the efficiency of the ciliary "escalator." Dried secretions are still a common cause of tube blockage and are the direct result of inadequate humidification. This, in turn, is usually the result of a failure to understand the principles of humidification or a failure to ensure that the principles are applied in the clinical situation. Tube blockage may not be seen with low levels of humidity when secretions are sparse, but failure to ensure adequate humidity in patients with a chest infection is a recipe for disaster.

The optimal humidity is obviously 43 g/m^3, but it is difficult to maintain this level continuously, and in clinical practice it has been found that secretions usually remain liquid when the humidity is maintained above 32 g/m^3. Further support for this figure has been provided by studies of ciliary activity which have shown that the rate of ciliary transport is not impaired when this minimum level of humidity is provided, though it was impaired when levels were reduced. The figure of 32 g/m^3 corresponds to a relative humidity of 100% at a temperature of 32°C, or 75% humidity at 37°C, and ciliary activity does not seem to be affected by temperatures between these two values providing that the minimum absolute value of humidity is maintained.[25,26] Ciliary activity seems to cease when the inspired gas temperature exceeds 41°C, and at higher temperatures there may be thermal damage to the trachea.[27] Humidification systems should therefore be fitted with safety devices that prevent the temperature at the patient connection port exceeding 41°C, even when the ventilator is temporarily disconnected.

Methods

Heat and moisture exchanger. The heat and moisture exchanger (HME) acts as an artificial nose, heat and moisture from the expired gas being retained on an element and the heat then being used to vaporise the condensed water during the next inspiration.[24] Early versions of this type of device used a metal gauze or foil element, but modern versions have an element made of paper or a special hydrophobic material. A recently introduced version incorporates a bacterial filter on the ventilator side of the humidity element, thus simplifying the breathing system still further.

The use of a HME obviates the risk of thermal damage to the trachea and possible infection from humidifers of the hot water type. Another advantage is that the breathing tubes remain dry. However, the device adds a small dead space and extra resistance to the breathing system, and the resistance of the element may be increased by droplets of mucopus. There have been many claims that HMEs have rendered other techniques of humidification obsolete, but most of the valid experimental studies suggest that water retention seldom exceeds 60% even under optimal conditions.

HMEs are of most value in patients who are ambulant and have a chronic tracheostomy. Such patients often have few secretions and are able to ensure patency of the tracheostomy tube with the aid of such a device, possibly augmented by occasional saline instillations. Exchangers may also be useful in patients with relatively normal lungs when short term ventilation is required—for example, during anaesthesia and the postoperative period; their use in patients with large amounts of secretions is, however, to be deprecated.

Instillation of saline. The regular injection of small aliquots of saline (2–10 ml in an adult) may be required to augment other methods if the patient has particularly tenacious secretions or if blood clots are present in the sputum. A slow intratracheal infusion of saline may be used as a method of humidification if other techniques are not available. The flow rate must be controlled with an infusion pump, or by infusion through a long narrow tube of appropriate resistance. The use of the standard infusion apparatus is fraught with danger because the drip control may be opened inadvertently, and the patient drowned. The drip rate should be adjusted to supply the volume of

195

saline required to humidify the patient's minute volume. For an adult breathing at 7 l/min this would amount to 0.043 ml × 7 = 0.3 ml/min.

Droplet humidifiers. Many types of humidifiers are designed to add droplets of water to the inspired gas. The droplets pass into the trachea and some are evaporated as the inspired gas is heated. Others are deposited on the walls of the trachea and major bronchi. The site of deposition depends on the size of the droplet and the velocity of air flow. Large droplets tend to deposit in the tubing leading to the patient; very small droplets are stable and are not deposited, though they may evaporate. Most of the droplets that deposit in the bronchi have a diameter of 1–10 microns.[28]

Most droplet humidifiers are driven by compressed gas. Water from a reservoir is sucked into a jet of gas and then impinges on a small sphere or anvil where it forms droplets. These are then passed through a baffle to remove the larger droplets before being transported to the patient. Another method of producing droplets is by directing a stream of water at a spinning disc. Very few of these devices produce enough droplets to produce full saturation of the air when this is heated to 37°C in the trachea.

Several extremely efficient ultrasonic devices were developed in the 1970s. These produced a dense cloud of droplets in the correct size range and had a small enough internal volume to be incorporated into the breathing system, but it was soon found that alveolar absorption of fluid tended to occur, and a number of patients suffered volume overload. In addition, lung lesions were reported in animals exposed to ultrasonic nebulisation and increases in airway resistance were reported in patients.[29] These devices are no longer used.

All forms of droplet humidifier suffer from the disadvantage that bacterial contamination in the water is transferred directly into the tracheobronchial tree.[30] Extreme care must be taken to maintain sterility by frequent sterilisation of the device and regular changes of water. Closed refilling systems require similar attention.

Hot water humidifers. Hot water humidifers provide the closest approximation to physiological conditions because they both warm and add vapour to the inspired gas. The earliest designs consisted of a metal chamber (about 30 cm square) partially filled with water. The water was heated to about 60°C by a thermostatically controlled electric kettle element, and the inspired gas picked up water vapour as it passed over the surface of the water. The surface area of the water was inadequate to produce full saturation of the gas, but as this passed along the ventilator tubing it cooled so that, although the absolute humidity was unchanged, the relative saturation increased to 100% and condensation occurred. By adjusting the temperature of the water in the can to produce a gas temperature of 32–37°C at the patient's end of the inspiratory tube adequate humidity could be maintained (fig 8.6).

This somewhat crude device had several disadvantages. Firstly, the

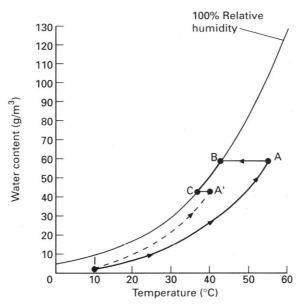

Fig 8.6 Principles of hot water humidification. Inspired gas (I) is assumed to be 30% saturated with water vapour at 10°C and contains about 3 g/m³ of water. Gas is warmed and moistened in the humidifer until it reaches (A). It then has a temperature of 55°C and a relative humidity of 60% (absolute humidity about 60 g/m³). Gas cools as it passes down the inspiratory tube and reaches (B) where the relative humidity is 100%. Further cooling results in condensation of the excess moisture within tube, gas finally reaching the patient at (C) with a temperature of 37°C and absolute humidity of 43 g/m³. Modern humidifiers have a larger vaporising surface and do not need to heat gas above 37-40°C to achieve adequate humidity. Furthermore, condensation in the breathing tube is often minimised by heating the tube. Humidification in such a device would follow the path 1←A'←C.

contacts of the thermostats tended to pit with the heavy electrical load of the heater element, so that temperature control was poor and thermostat failure was common. Secondly, the temperature at the patient depended on both the heat transmitted to the gas in the tank and the subsequent cooling as it passed along the inspiratory tube. If the flow rate in the inspiratory tube increased, as it did when the patient was temporarily disconnected from a pressure generator type of ventilator such as the East-Radcliffe, the temperature at the patient's end of the tube increased abruptly. The hot gas could then damage the trachea when the patient was reconnected. The risk could be reduced by decreasing the heat loss along the tube by lagging or by using a flow generator type of ventilator, but the system was obviously unsatisfactory.

Modern hot water humidifiers incorporate a number of improvements. The chamber containing the water is reduced in size so that the compressed gas volume is small. The water temperature is kept close to 37°C, eliminating the risk of delivering dangerously hot gas when flow rate is increased. Full

197

Improvements in hot water humidifiers

- Small internal gas volume
- Water temperature maintained close to 37°C
- Full saturation of gas leaving chamber
- Cooling in inspiratory tube minimised
- Gas pathway and water chamber removable for sterilisation
- Water level maintained automatically
- Audible and visual alarms indicate malfunction

---

saturation of the gas leaving the chamber is assured by increasing the water surface area by means of a wick. Cooling of gas in the inspiratory tube is prevented by heating the tube with a heating wire, the temperature of the wire being servocontrolled from a temperature sensor at the patient's end of the delivery tube.

These humidifiers have several other advantages. The water chamber is usually heated by a thermostatically controlled hotplate and can be removed for sterilisation or can be replaced by one of smaller volume for neonatal or paediatric use. The correct water level can be maintained by an automatic device connected directly to sterile infusion bags, and audible and visual alarms are provided to indicate malfunction.

Some humidifers do not have these refinements. Many can be used with safety providing that they are used with careful monitoring of the inspired gas temperature. In some hot water humidifiers the gas is bubbled under the surface of the water in an attempt to increase the humidity. This greatly increases the inspiratory resistance, which may not matter when the patient is being ventilated mechanically but can impose a severe increase in the work of breathing when a spontaneous breathing mode is used.

Removal of secretions

In patients with an artificial airway, secretion removal is impaired because the normal ciliary escalator is interrupted by the presence of a cuffed tube, and its effectiveness is reduced by the presence of thick secretions. Adequate hydration is therefore a keynote of treatment. Of even more importance is the absence of the normal expulsive cough mechanism. These problems are overcome by transferring secretions to the major airways by postural drainage and physiotherapy, from which they can be removed by blind tracheobronchial suction or bronchoscopy.

Postural drainage

Secretions from localised areas of lung disease can be encouraged to drain into the trachea by nursing the patient in a position that promotes good postural drainage (fig 8.7). When the disease is more widespread the patient should be turned every hour or two.

Physiotherapy

Physiotherapy with manual percussion over the affected zones can help to remove secretions from the periphery to the central airways. This treatment may increase bronchospasm, so it may be advisable to pretreat the patient with inhaled bronchodilators.

The most effective way of moving secretions in the absence of the natural cough is the technique of assisted coughing. This can be performed while the patient is being mechanically ventilated but is most effective if performed with manually controlled ventilation. The lung is hyperinflated and the pressure on the reservoir bag is suddenly released. The release of pressure is timed to coincide with an expiratory squeeze and vibration of the chest wall produced by the physiotherapist. The procedure is carried out rhythmically at a rate of about 20 breaths a minute, and each area of the chest is treated in turn. Usually, secretions can be heard in the main bronchi after 5–10 breaths and the procedure is then interrupted while they are aspirated. If there are obvious areas of collapse and the secretions are viscid it is helpful to instill aliquots of saline with the affected area in a dependent position. The patient is then turned so that this area is uppermost and expiratory vibration and percussion performed.

The hyperinflations used in this form of physiotherapy may result in a decrease in cardiac output, particularly if the patient has a low blood volume or an unstable cardiovascular system. The decrease in output results in a decrease in mixed venous PO_2 that tends to offset the effects of any reduction in venous admixture on arterial PO_2. Beneficial effects of physiotherapy on gas exchange may therefore not appear until cardiac output has returned to normal levels. The frequency and duration of this type of physiotherapy must be tailored carefully to the patient's condition.

Bronchial lavage

Bronchial lavage has been advocated as a method of clearing secretions in patients with severe asthma or with alveolar proteinosis, but can also be valuable in patients with viscid secretions and areas of collapse. It is usually performed by injecting saline into each of the segmental bronchi in turn under bronchoscopic control.

Conclusions

An artificial airway bypasses the protective and conditioning mechanisms normally provided by the upper airway, so that these must be replaced by

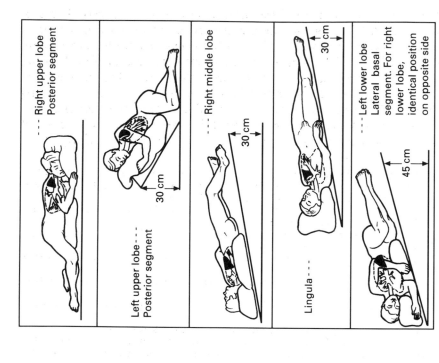

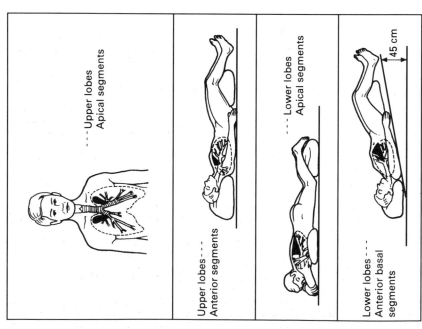

Fig 8.7 Positions for postural drainage.

artificial devices. Since the airway itself is in contact with body tissues, it must be made of biologically inert materials and so designed that it has a minimal effect on the surfaces with which it is in contact. Although modern technology has resulted in many improvements in the design of tracheal and tracheostomy tubes, their use is still associated with a high incidence of complications, especially those associated with pressure on the surrounding tissues, and wound and chest infection. Since these complications may compromise survival, every effort must be made to use techniques of respiratory support that do not require the use of an artificial airway.

1 Asai T, Vaughan RS. Misuse of the laryngeal mask airway. *Anaesthesia* 1994;**49**:467–9.
2 Aebert H, Hunefeld G, Regal G. Paranasal sinusitis and sepsis in ICU patients with nasotracheal intubation. *Intensive Care Med* 1988;**15**:27–30.
3 Jones R, Bodnar A, Roan Y, Johnson D. Subglottic stenosis in newborn intensive care unit graduates. *Am J Dis Child* 1981;**135**:367–8.
4 Dankle SK, Schuller DE, McClead RE. Prolonged intubation of neonates. *Arch Otolaryngol Head Neck Surg* 1987;**113**:841–3.
5 Leigh JM, Maynard JP. Pressure on the tracheal mucosa from cuffed tubes. *BMJ* 1979;**i**: 1173–4.
6 Macrea W. Wallace P. Aspiration around high-volume low-pressure endotracheal cuff. *BMJ* 1981;**283**:1220.
7 Crawley BE, Cross DE. Tracheal cuffs. A review and dynamic pressure study. *Anaesthesia* 1975;**30**:4–11.
8 Wee MYK. The oesophageal detector device. *Anaesthesia* 1988;**43**:27–9.
9 Brunel W, Coleman DL, Schwartz DE, Peper E, Cohen NH. Assessment of routine chest roentgenograms and the physical examination to confirm endotracheal tube position. *Chest* 1989;**96**:1043–5.
10 Rivera R, Tibballs J. Complications of endotracheal intubation and mechanical ventilation in infants and children. *Crit Care Med* 1992;**20**:193–9.
11 Kastanos N, Estopá Miro R, Marin Perez A, Xaubet Mir A, Agusti-Vidal A. Laryngotracheal injury due to endotracheal intubation: incidence, evolution, and predisposing factors. A prospective long-term study. *Crit Care Med* 1983;**11**:362–7.
12 Stauffer JL, Olson DE, Petty TL. Complications and consequences of endotracheal intubation and tracheostomy. A prospective study of 150 critically ill patients. *Am J Med* 1981;**70**:65–75.
13 Stock MC, Woodward CG, Shapiro BA, Cane RD, Lewis V, Pecaro B. Perioperative complications of elective tracheostomy in critically ill patients. *Crit Care Med* 1986;**14**:861–3.
14 Heffner JE. Timing of tracheotomy in mechanically ventilated patients. *Am Rev Respir Dis* 1993;**147**:768–71.
15 Colice GL, Stukel TA, Dain B. Laryngeal complications of prolonged intubation. *Chest* 1989;**96**:877–84.
16 Dunham CM, LaMonica C. Prolonged tracheal intubation in the trauma patient. *J Trauma* 1984;**24**:120–4.
17 King TA, Adams AP. Failed tracheal intubation. *Br J Anaesth* 1990;**65**:400–14.
18 Matthews HR, Hopkinson RB. Treatment of sputum retention by mini-tracheotomy. *Br J Surg* 1984;**71**:147–50.
19 Jackson IJB, Choudhry AK, Ryan DW, Matthews HR, Corke CF. Minitracheotomy Seldinger—assessment of a new technique. *Anaesthesia* 1991;**46**:475–7.
20 Ryan DW. Minitracheotomy. *Intensive Care World* 1991;**8**:128–31.
21 Griggs WM, Worthley LIG, Gilligan JE, Thomas PD, Myburg JA. A simple percutaneous tracheostomy technique. *Surg Gynec Obstet* 1990;**170**:543–5.
22 Griggs WM, Myburg JA. Worthley LIG. A prospective comparison of a percutaneous tracheostomy technique with standard tracheostomy. *Intensive Care Med* 1991;**17**:261–3.
23 Heffner JE. Percutaneous tracheostomy—novel technique or technical novelty? *Intensive Care Med* 1991;**17**:252–3.

24 Hedley RM. Allt-Graham J. Heat and moisture exchangers and breathing filters. *Br J Anaesth* 1994;**73**:227–36.
25 Forbes AR. Humidification and mucus flow in the intubated trachea. *Br J Anaesth* 1973; **45**:874–8.
26 Forbes AR. Temperature, humidity and mucus flow in the intubated trachea. *Br J Anaesth* 1974;**46**:29–34.
27 Dahlhamn T. Mucous flow and ciliary activity in the trachea of healthy rats and rats exposed to respiratory irritant gases. *Acta Physiol Scand* 1956;**36**(suppl 123):1–161.
28 Morrow PE. Aerosol characterization and deposition. *Am Rev Respir Dis* 1974;**110**:88–99.
29 Cheney FW, Butler J. The effects of ultrasonically produced aerosols on airway resistance in man. *Anesthesiology* 1968;**29**:1099–106.
30 Moffet HL, Allan D, Williams T. Survival and dissemination of bacteria in nebulizers and incubators. *Am J Dis Child* 1967;**114**:13–20.

9 Care of the patient during respiratory support

The indications for the provision of respiratory support and the choice of airway have been discussed in chapters 7 and 8. The following sections deal with the choice of support mode and the initiation of support, the general care of the patient, and the problems of weaning.

Choice of support mode

The guiding principle in choosing the mode of support is to use the minimum amount of support necessary to provide adequate oxygenation of the tissues. Secondary considerations are maintaining a reasonable acid-base status and the comfort of the patient. In patients with very severe ARDS, oxygen availability may be increased by producing complete apnoea and so reducing oxygen consumption to a minimum. Complete control of ventilation may also be desirable in patients with head injuries, in those requiring therapeutic use of the muscle relaxant drugs, and in those with respiratory centre depression. In most other patients there are advantages in maintaining a spontaneous respiratory component during respiratory support.

Non-invasive methods

The first step is to decide whether the patient could benefit from any of the non-invasive methods of support such as mask CPAP, negative pressure ventilation, or nasal intermittent positive pressure ventilation (see chapter 10). For a given level of positive end expiratory pressure CPAP produces a greater increase in FRC than controlled ventilation with PEEP.[1] Since it also results in the least increase in intrathoracic pressure for a given increase in lung volume and may decrease the work of breathing,[2] it is worth using CPAP as the first line of treatment in patients with pulmonary congestion or oedema due to left ventricular failure,[3] in those suspected of developing ARDS, and in patients with pneumonia.[4]

Mask CPAP is valuable in helping to splint the chest wall in patients with chest trauma and it improves oxygenation when there is pulmonary contusion. It is also useful in treating *Pneumocystis carinii* pneumonia.[5] Applying CPAP by nasal mask may produce a dramatic improvement in patients who have episodes of obstructive sleep apnoea, particularly if these complicate an acute respiratory infection or are a pulmonary complication of operation. Nasal intermittent positive pressure ventilation may help those with borderline respiratory failure that is worsened by sleep. It may also prove valuable in providing support to patients with limited respiratory reserve during an exacerbation of acute lung disease. Negative pressure ventilation is also helpful in this category of patient, but its successful application depends on the ability of the patient to maintain a patent airway, especially when the pharyngeal muscles are relaxed by sleep.

Controlled mechanical ventilation

If non-invasive methods are no longer appropriate, it is necessary to intubate the trachea. In some centres this is effected with topical anaesthesia with or without sedation, but usually the tube is inserted under intravenous anaesthesia with a muscle relaxant drug. This enables the ventilation to be controlled at an appropriate level, provides an opportunity for physiotherapy and bronchial toilet with a suction catheter or bronchoscope, and also enables analgesia to be established without risk of respiratory depression. It is likely that the tidal volume and frequency will have been selected by the anaesthetist on the basis of blood gas results, and a decision will have been taken concerning the most desirable PCO_2 and PO_2 levels. In most patients the aim will be to keep PCO_2 and PO_2 within normal limits. However, PCO_2 should initially be maintained close to preintubation values in patients who have had a chronically increased PCO_2, for a rapid reduction of PCO_2 may lead to a reduction in cardiac output and hypotension, particularly if the patient is dehydrated. Patients with chronic CO_2 retention have high concentrations of bicarbonate in plasma and cerebrospinal fluid and may develop severe cerebral vasoconstriction when PCO_2 is lowered rapidly; this may lead to convulsions, grand mal epilepsy, and lasting cerebral damage.[6]

Other patients with a non-respiratory disturbance of acid-base balance may also require PCO_2 to be maintained at an abnormal level in order to keep the arterial pH within reasonable limits. In such patients the pH rather than the PCO_2 should determine the level of ventilatory support provided. In patients with ARDS and asthma there is an increasing tendency to maintain PCO_2 at higher than normal levels. This increases the quantity of CO_2 eliminated per unit volume of ventilation and enables tidal volumes and peak airway pressures to be reduced in patients with a low compliance or high airway resistance.[7]

In most patients with relatively normal lungs it is reasonable to choose a tidal volume in the range of 10–15 ml/kg and to ventilate at a frequency of 10–12 breaths/min. If PEEP is added, tidal volume should be reduced to 8–12 ml/kg to reduce peak airway pressure. Further reductions in tidal volume may be necessary if lung compliance is less than 0.30–0.35 l/kPa. If tidal volume is reduced it may be necessary to increase respiratory frequency to 15–20 breaths/min in order to maintain adequate alveolar ventilation. If this is done, regular checks should be made to ensure that intrinsic PEEP is not developing. Many believe that the use of the pressure generator mode or pressure cycling is advantageous in this situation to ensure that the ventilated areas of lung are not overdistended. Since resistance and compliance may change rapidly, careful monitoring of expired tidal volume (with due allowance for the internal compliance of the breathing system) is essential.

Some ventilators have a sigh function which delivers a tidal volume approximately double the set volume every 100 breaths. This is a heritage from the 1960s, when it was suggested that a regular sigh prevented atelectasis in patients with a reduced lung volume, but subsequent studies have not provided any evidence that it improves lung function.

Controlled ventilation with positive end expiratory pressure

The patient will usually have received a high inspired oxygen concentration during the intubation or tracheostomy, and this may need to be reduced towards the 50% concentration that is generally regarded as the safe maximum for chronic exposure.[8] In patients with a large increase in intrapulmonary shunt this concentration may not relieve arterial hypoxaemia. In such circumstances it may be necessary to add a positive end expiratory pressure to increase lung volume and decrease shunt.

There have been many suggestions concerning the best method of choosing the optimal level of PEEP, and there is still a wide variation in practice between different centres. One of the first studies on this subject was that carried out by Suter and colleagues. They found that increasing levels of PEEP produced a progressive decrease in shunt and increase in arterial PO_2. However, there was a decrease in cardiac output at the higher levels of PEEP. The net result was that increasing levels of PEEP initially produced an increase in oxygen transport, but this reached a maximum and then decreased again at the higher levels of PEEP. They found that the highest level of oxygen transport occurred at the PEEP level at which total thoracic compliance was maximal and so suggested that this measurement could be used to determine what they termed "best PEEP." They also found that dead space/tidal volume ratio was least at this level.[9] Unfortunately others have not been able to confirm the relation between compliance and oxygen delivery.[10] It has also been suggested that the optimal PEEP level may correspond with the point at which the arterial to end tidal PCO_2 difference is minimal,[11] but the value of this technique has not been confirmed.[12]

Another more practical suggestion is to set the PEEP level at the pressure corresponding to the inflection point on the inspiratory limb of the pressure-volume curve.[13] This point seems to define the pressure level at which a high proportion of alveolar units reopen and corresponds to the pressure level which also results in a significant reduction in shunt (see fig 2.12). However, such an inflection point is usually present only in patients with pulmonary oedema and in the early stages of ARDS, so the method has a limited sphere of application. The inflection point may also be due to the presence of intrinsic PEEP.

Another group has suggested that much higher (optimal) levels of PEEP are required in patients with severe lung disease. They have claimed that "optimal" PEEP levels of up to 44 cm H_2O could be tolerated without a decrease in cardiac output when the ventilation was being supported by IMV.[14] However, subsequent studies have shown that such high levels of PEEP frequently result in barotrauma and may decrease oxygen delivery,[15] and it is now clear that the phase of applying very high PEEP levels to secure maximal lung inflation is over. Since the only prospective, randomised trials of the use of PEEP suggest that the application of PEEP is associated with an increase in mortality,[16,17] it would seem logical to use a PEEP level that is the minimal compatible with an adequate supply of oxygen to the tissues. This can be determined only by measuring cardiac output and arterial oxygen content. However, if such measurements cannot be made it would seem reasonable to optimise cardiac output by cautious fluid loading or the use of a low dose infusion of an inotrope, or both, and then to increase the PEEP level in increments of 3–5 cm H_2O until an arterial PO_2 of 8–9 kPa (60–70 mm Hg) is achieved on an inspired oxygen concentration of 50–60%. When PEEP is applied the peak inflation pressure will rise, so increasing the risk of barotrauma.[18] In patients with ARDS the lowest compliance is found at high and low tidal volumes,[19] so tidal volumes should be reduced to 5–10 ml/kg when a PEEP of 8–12 cm H_2O is being used in order to keep the tidal volume on the steep part of the pressure-volume curve.[20]

Choice of spontaneous breathing mode

The decrease in cardiac output resulting from the use of any technique that increases mean airway pressure can be minimised with a ventilatory mode that incorporates a spontaneous breathing component. Spontaneous ventilation may improve the distribution of ventilation and may prevent disuse atrophy of the respiratory muscles.[21] It also reduces the need for sedation. On the other hand, it increases the work of breathing and so may increase oxygen consumption. Inadequate respiratory support may result in respiratory muscle fatigue, tachypnoea, respiratory distress, and patient discomfort, and this may prolong the period of weaning.

Assisted ventilation delivers a preset pattern of breath whenever the ventilator mechanism is triggered by the patient. Most patients find this less

Spontaneous breathing modes

Advantages
  Less risk of pulmonary barotrauma
  Decreased mean intrathoracic pressure
    Decrease in cardiac output minimised
    Improved renal function
  Decreased requirement for sedation
  Patient can set PCO_2 levels
  Preservation of respiratory muscle function
  Possibly improved gas distribution in lungs

Disadvantages
  Increased work of breathing: may increase oxygen consumption and cause fatigue
  Require efficient patient triggering devices if synchronised
  Require sophisticated monitoring systems
  PCO_2 level set by patient may be inappropriate

acceptable than inspiratory pressure support so the assisted mode is now rarely used. Most units now use ventilators that can provide intermittent mandatory ventilation (IMV), synchronised intermittent mandatory ventilation (SIMV), mandatory minute volume (MMV), or inspiratory pressure support (IPS) modes. All can be used with PEEP so that an adequate lung volume is maintained with both spontaneous and mandatory breaths and oxygenation is not compromised by the relatively low frequency of mandatory breaths.

SIMV has theoretical advantages over IMV since it is designed to reduce the "stacking" of breaths that might be expected to occur if a mandatory breath were to be delivered synchronously with a spontaneous breath, but this stacking does not seem to be a serious problem. Both IMV and SIMV require careful adjustment of the frequency and characteristics of the mandatory breath to ensure that adequate ventilatory assistance is being provided, but both modes are flexible and combine spontaneous ventilation with a guaranteed minimum minute ventilation. Many ventilators now enable inspiratory pressure support to be added to the spontaneous breaths when SIMV is engaged.

The MMV mode provides additional ventilatory support (usually in the form of extra mandatory breaths) if the patient fails to achieve a preset minute volume with spontaneous breathing. The patient may, however, generate a minute volume greater than that set on the machine with an inefficient pattern of fast, shallow breathing and so may not receive any mechanical assistance, even though the alveolar ventilation is grossly deficient. Another disadvantage of the technique is that it is difficult to predict what minute volume a patient actually requires. Metabolic rate

207

fluctuates with the movements of the patient, and the work of breathing and ratio of dead space to tidal volume depend on the type of ventilation (spontaneous or controlled) and on tidal volume and respiratory frequency.

With some of the earlier systems it was not possible for the patient to increase the minute volume above the set MMV level. However, the extended MMV (EMMV) mode on the Engström Elvira permits the patient to inspire more than the set MMV, as does the minimum minute volume mode on the Dräger Evita ventilator. The MMV mode on the Hamilton Veolar differs from that on the other ventilators for it measures the patient's spontaneous breathing over a period of eight breaths and then continuously adjusts the level of inspiratory pressure support to maintain the set MMV. Thus the pressure support may be reduced if the patient exceeds the set level.

The inspiratory pressure support (IPS) mode seems to have several advantages over the other spontaneous breathing modes. Each breath is supported to an extent which enables the patient to achieve an adequate tidal volume so that the patient should have complete control of the breath pattern and frequency of breathing. Support can be varied between almost complete support, which can abolish most of the work of breathing, to a low level of support, which just replaces the work performed against the extra resistances encountered when breathing through a tracheal tube and ventilator system. This should enable the respiratory muscles to work with optimal efficiency, prevent fatigue, and facilitate weaning.[22]

In practice, however, there are often difficulties with patient triggering,[23] and it is difficult to know what level of support to provide. The correct level of support should enable the patient to breathe with a normal tidal volume and frequency. It should shorten inspiratory time and so allow more time for expiration.[24] If the support level is too low the patient will develop shallow tidal volumes and tachypnoea, but if it is set too high the patient's respiratory drive may be decreased and apnoea may occur. This may be dangerous if the ventilator has no back up mandatory ventilation mode to maintain a basal level of support. Although a back up mode is available on some machines, it may have to be switched on specially when the inspiratory support mode is engaged. Yet another disadvantage of the technique is that mean intrathoracic pressure is usually higher than with techniques that allow a number of unassisted breaths between mandatory breaths. For these reasons many units prefer to use SIMV with moderate pressure support of the spontaneous breaths.

With all these spontaneous breathing modes it is important to observe the frequency and pattern of spontaneous breathing and to adjust the ventilatory support to a level that provides the most natural pattern and frequency of spontaneous breathing. Frequent blood gas measurements are also required in the early stages of treatment. Activity in the sternomastoid muscle suggests that the patient is using the accessory muscles of respiration and is a further sign that respiratory support should be increased.

Other modes

The use of the more specialised modes designed specifically to reduce peak airway pressure (see chapter 5) is more controversial. Inverse ratio ventilation (IRV) is often tried when high levels of PEEP fail to improve oxygenation. Its main advantage is that it allows ventilation to be reduced by about 10%, so it can help to reduce peak airway pressure. Some workers claim that it also improves oxygenation, but as its use is associated with an increase in mean airway pressure this may decrease cardiac output so that oxygen delivery is not improved.

The technique of airway pressure release ventilation (APRV), in which spontaneous breathing at a high CPAP level is periodically interrupted by allowing the patient to expire to a lower PEEP level for 1–2 seconds, has been used successfully in patients with moderately severe lung disease. It provides a pattern of lung volume change similar to inverse ratio ventilation and therefore reduces peak pressures, but it allows the patient to continue breathing spontaneously. The spontaneous breathing component may increase cardiac output[25] and improve ventilation distribution[26] when compared with controlled ventilation but may also increase the work of breathing.

Biphasic positive airway pressure breathing (BIPAP) enables the patient's spontaneous breathing levels to be cycled between high and low PEEP levels with varying inspiratory and expiratory times and would seem to have similar effects to the use of the pressure generator mode, except that there is a superimposed spontaneous component. Although the retention of spontaneous breathing may reduce the need for sedation and should minimise mean intrathoracic pressure, there have been no studies comparing the short and long term effects of BIPAP with a similar pattern of controlled ventilation.

As discussed in chapter 5, there now seem to be few indications for the use of high frequency ventilation. High frequency jet ventilation may be considered in patients with a large bronchopleural fistula, for there is some evidence that it may reduce the air leak, even if it does not decrease mortality, and there are a few anaesthetic indications for its use. High frequency chest wall oscillation increases CO_2 elimination in patients with acute or chronic lung disease but is still being evaluated. Extracorporeal membrane oxygenation has a definite place in treating respiratory insufficiency in neonates, but there is still no proof that extracorporeal CO_2 removal reduces mortality in adults with severe respiratory distress.

Care of the patient on respiratory support

Treatment in an intensive care unit is a frightening experience and many of the procedures, such as catheterisation, the insertion of a chest drain, the changing of surgical dressings, or turning may be painful. There is a continual background of noise and activity, and the normal diurnal rhythms are disturbed by the need for continuous observation and treatment. Sleep deprivation is therefore almost inevitable. Careful adjustment of alarm settings and the behaviour of staff around the patient can do much to reduce noise levels and sleep disturbance. Discomfort can be minimised by frequent changes in position, careful adjustment of the position of ventilator and drainage tubing, and frequent skin and mouth care. Anxiety can be reduced by informing the patient before undertaking any monitoring or therapeutic activity and by continually updating the patient on progress. It is important to minimise disorientation in time by reducing lighting levels at night whenever possible, encouraging contact with the outside world by the provision of a television or radio, and ensuring that the patient receives frequent visits from relatives who have been kept fully informed about his or her condition. Attention to these details can reduce the need for analgesia and sedation. The use of scoring systems for anxiety and pain can also help to make staff aware of the problems. Even so, most patients will require sedation and analgesia at some stage during their stay in an intensive care unit.

Patients who are disorientated, and those who have suffered severe trauma or head injuries, will usually require heavy sedation or even muscle paralysis to enable ventilation to be controlled. A similar level of sedation and, possibly, paralysis may also be required to control tetanic spasms and to reduce oxygen consumption in patients with ARDS or septic shock. In most other cases requiring respiratory support sedation may be minimised to permit the adoption of spontaneous breathing modes, and pain relief may be required only for specific causes such as wound pain or the discomfort caused by a tracheal tube.

Analgesia, sedation, and paralysis

Analgesics. Pain relief is usually achieved by repeated bolus doses or infusions of an opiate such as morphine. Bolus doses have the disadvantage that the blood level fluctuates above and below the optimal therapeutic level, but the use of infusions may result in overdosage. If an infusion is preceded by a bolus dose, and the infusion rate is then carefully controlled on the basis of pain scoring, very satisfactory results can be achieved.

In many patients, patient controlled analgesia provides an excellent alternative. The patient is connected to a computer controlled syringe containing 60 ml of morphine 1–2 mg/ml and the device set to deliver a bolus of 1 mg on demand with a lockout period of, say, 5–10 minutes. If necessary, an antiemetic such as droperidol 0.05 mg/ml may be added to minimise nausea. Most patients soon develop confidence in their ability to control pain

Analgesics and respiratory support

Morphine
- Inexperience
- But—Dilates venous system; may cause hypotension
  Depresses respiration and cough reflex; maty hinder weaning
  Depresses gastric emptying and gut motility; may delay enteral feeding
  Tolerance may occur
  Action may be prolonged in patients with kidney and liver problems

Fentanyl
- Short duration of bolus is due to redistribution rather than clearance

Alfentanil
- Short elimination half life; suitable for continuous infusion
  Eliminated by hepatic metabolism

Non-steroidal anti-inflammatory drugs
- May be given orally or rectally
  May produce clotting abnormalities, gastrointestinal bleeding, renal failure

50/50 nitrous oxide/oxygen (Entonox)
- Useful for short, painful procedures

and learn to press the button in anticipation of a painful event. The technique is particularly helpful in patients who would otherwise fear moving around because of pain from a surgical wound.

Morphine is cheap but has some disadvantages. It dilates the venous system and will tend to cause hypotension if the patient's legs are dependent or the blood volume is reduced. It depresses respiration and the cough reflex, which may prove useful in some circumstances but may hinder weaning. Morphine also depresses gastric emptying and gut motility and may delay enteral feeding. Tolerance to the drug may occur, but addiction is unlikely if it is used to relieve pain. The elimination of active morphine metabolites is delayed in patients with renal impairment and this may cause prolonged action of the drug.[27] Liver failure may also impair morphine metabolism.[28]

Shorter acting drugs such as fentanyl and alfentanil also have disadvantages. A single bolus dose of fentanyl has a short duration of action, but this is due to redistribution rather than clearance, so the drug should not be given as an infusion. Alfentanil has a short elimination half life and a small volume of distribution and is therefore suitable for continuous infusion. However, it is eliminated by hepatic metabolism.[29]

Non-steroidal anti-inflammatory drugs such as indomethacin may also prove valuable in relieving pain of an inflammatory nature. They may be given orally or rectally and reduce opioid requirements after operation. However, they may produce clotting abnormalities, gastrointestinal bleeding, and renal failure.

211

Sedatives and respiratory support

Benzodiazepines
    Produce amnesia and decrease in muscle tone

Diazepam
    Active metabolites have long half life
    Tends to produce venous thrombosis

Midazolam
    Can be used as infusion
    Action is sometimes prolonged in patients with multiple organ failure

Chlormethiazole
    Can be used as infusion
    Good anticonvulsant
    Recovery is slow
    Large fluid load

Propofol
    Depth of sedation is easily adjusted
    Recovery is extremely rapid
    Expensive
    High lipid load may increase CO_2 production

Isoflurane
    Pollution problems
    Accumulation of fluoride ions may lead to renal failure
    Expensive

Regional analgesia. Regional analgesic techniques are being increasingly used for pain relief where the site of the pain is well defined. Bolus doses or infusions of local anaesthetic drugs may be given by the epidural route and may be supplemented by epidural opiates. Although epidural opiates add a small risk of delayed respiratory depression, this is of less concern when the patient is being nursed with full monitoring in an intensive care unit than when being nursed on the general wards.

Sedation. The most commonly used sedative drugs are the benzodiazepines, but they do not produce analgesia and must be combined with the opioids if pain is present. They also produce amnesia and a decrease in muscle tone. Diazepam has active metabolites with a long half life and tends to produce venous thrombosis. It is therefore unsuitable for use in intravenous infusions. Midazolam has an elimination half life of 2–4 hours after a bolus dose and is suitable for use as an infusion. However, it sometimes has a prolonged action in patients with multiple organ failure. Another drug which is used for sedation is chlormethiazole. This can be used as in infusion and is a good anticonvulsant, though recovery is slow and the fluid load may prove excessive.[30]

212

Muscle relaxants and respiratory support

Suxamethonium
    May lead to hyperkalaemia
    Increases intraocular pressure
    May produce bradycardia

Pancuronium, vecuronium
    Excretion may be delayed by hepatic or renal impairment

Atracurium
    Metabolite has central excitatory effects
    Accumulates in patients with renal failure

Propofol infusions are being increasingly used in intensive care, for the depth of sedation is easily adjusted and recovery is extremely rapid. Because of the cost many units reserve propofol sedation for situations where rapid recovery is required, for example, in patients with head injury who may require repeated assessment. The high lipid load may also be important, for it increases CO_2 production.

Inhalation anaesthetics have also been used for sedation. Many years ago nitrous oxide was used to sedate patients with tetanus, but this led to megaloblastic anaemia. The use of 50/50 oxygen/nitrous oxide mixture (Entonox) is now restricted to providing pain relief for short procedures such as drain removal or physiotherapy in patients with fractured ribs. Low concentrations of isoflurane have also been advocated for sedation and pain relief,[31] but the pollution problems, the possibility of renal failure from the accumulation of fluoride ions, and the cost implications have prevented the widespread adoption of this technique.[32]

Muscle relaxants. The use of muscle relaxants in the intensive care unit has decreased greatly in recent years.[33] Suxamethonium is the only depolarising muscle relaxant in common use; because of its short action, it is often used for intubation. Suxamethonium releases potassium from muscles and considerable hyperkalaemia may occur after injection in patients with burns (3 weeks to 3 months), stroke, spinal cord damage, Duchenne's muscular dystrophy, and severe intra-abdominal infection. It is contraindicated in patients with an eye injury because it increases intraocular pressure. It may also produce bradycardia, particularly if more than one dose has been given, and histamine release.

The most commonly used longer acting non-depolarising agents are pancuronium, vecuronium, and atracurium. The excretion of pancuronium and vecuronium may be delayed by hepatic or renal impairment. Atracurium is metabolised to laudanosine, which has central excitatory effects and accumulates in patients with renal failure.[34]

Nutrition

The nutrition of the patient tends to be ignored during the first few days of intensive care treatment, but it should be included in any treatment plan, for variations in metabolism can add considerably to the CO_2 load. The energy requirements of patients in intensive care may be calculated by determining the basal metabolic rate from tables of body weight or surface area and then adding increments to allow for the increased metabolism associated with the disease process.[35] Thus a 50 kg woman might have a basal metabolic rate of 6250 kJ (1500 kcal)/day whereas an 80 kg man might have a rate of 10 000 kJ (2400 kcal)/day. This requirement might be increased by 5–10% in patients after operation, by 25% in those with peritonitis and by 50–70% in those with severe burns. A further 20% increase might be required if the patient was not sedated and had an increased work of breathing. These estimates provide a relatively inaccurate guide to total energy consumption, and many units are now investing in indirect calorimetry equipment that allows the energy requirements to be measured directly, whether the patient is breathing spontaneously or is connected to a ventilator.

The basic principle is that the CO_2 output and O_2 consumption are calculated from the difference in gas concentrations between inspired and expired gas. Since there is no CO_2 in inspired gas, the CO_2 output is the product of the mixed expired concentration and the expired volume, both of which can be measured easily. The O_2 consumption is calculated from the difference between the inspired and expired volumes of oxygen. The expired volume of O_2 can be calculated from the mixed expired concentration and expired volume, but as the inspired volume cannot be measured with accuracy it is calculated from the expired volume by applying the "Haldane correction." This utilises the difference in nitrogen concentration between inspired and expired gas (calculated by subtracting the sum of the O_2 and CO_2 concentrations from unity) to indicate how much shrinkage of alveolar gas has been produced by the different volumes of O_2 and CO_2 exchanged.

To ensure an acceptable degree of accuracy (an error of less than 10%) the inspired oxygen concentration must be accurately controlled throughout the period of measurement; there must be a leakproof circuit; and gas concentrations must be analysed with a high degree of precision. Several commercially available devices now have an acceptable accuracy.[36,37]

The values for CO_2 output and O_2 consumption provide a measure of energy consumption and allow the respiratory quotient (RQ = CO_2 output ÷ O_2 consumption) to be calculated. Carbohydrate has an RQ of 1.0, fat 0.7, protein 0.82, and lipogenesis (the synthesis of fat from glucose) 0.8. If carbohydrates are given in excess of the energy consumption there will be excess lipogenesis and an increase in CO_2 load. This will require an unnecessarily high level of ventilation to maintain a normal PCO_2 and may prevent weaning. To correct this the proportion of carbohydrates to calories not containing nitrogen should be reduced to 40–60% and the rest given as fat.

Other care

Care of the lungs. In the intubated patient regular turning from side to side (and into the prone position, if tolerated) helps to maintain lung expansion and aids drainage of secretions. Secretion removal can be expedited by regular sessions of manual hyperinflation of the lungs, with external chest vibration and compression during each expiration. This is a highly effective method of expelling secretions but should be used with care in patients with haemodynamic instability. Suction catheters should be passed with a "no touch" technique. Disposable sealed units facilitate this procedure. Catheters should be manufactured from a non-irritant material, should have an end hole and at least one side hole, and should be used with the minimal effective suction pressure to minimise tracheal mucosal damage. The external diameter of the catheter should be less than one half of the internal diameter of the tracheal or tracheostomy tube so as to prevent the generation of a subatmospheric pressure within the lungs.

If atelectasis develops, it may prove helpful to instil 5–10 ml aliquots of saline into the main bronchus on the side of the collapse and then to use postural drainage to encourage secretions to drain from the affected area. If a localised area of collapse does not respond to vigorous physiotherapy and postural drainage, fibreoptic bronchoscopy and suction should be used to clear secretions from the appropriate bronchus.

Preventing other complications. There have been several excellent reviews of the inumerable complications associated with mechanical support.[38,39] Although many complications can be prevented, there is still no general agreement concerning the most effective ways of reducing the incidence of some of the most serious complications such as infection, pulmonary embolus, and gastrointestinal bleeding.

Secondary chest infection is common in any patient with an artificial airway and is particularly dangerous in the immunocompromised patient. Infection may originate in the apparatus attached to the patient or may be transmitted to the patient by the attending staff. However, there is now much evidence to suggest that in many cases the infection is due to bacteria carried by the patient. Unfortunately, many of these infections are resistant to standard antibiotics. This has led to attempts to eliminate the source of infection by selective decontamination of the gut with massive doses of wide spectrum antibiotics. Despite many studies, there is no clear evidence to suggest that this expensive approach to the problem is cost effective.[40]

Another of the major problems resulting from immobility is the prevention of venous thrombosis and pulmonary embolism. The venous circulation can

---

Major complications associated with mechanical ventialtion

Pulmonary
  Associated with artificial airway
  Pulmonary barotrauma
  Chest infection
  Venous thrombosis and pulmonary embolism
  Lung fibrosis (late)

Cardiovascular
  Decreased cardiac output and hypotension
  Dysrhythmias
  Pulmonary artery catheter complications

Gastrointestinal
  Pneumoperitoneum
  Decreased gastrointestinal motility
  Gastrointestinal haemorrhage

Nutritional
  Malnutrition
  Metabolic
  Excess CO_2 production

Renal
  Fluid retention
  Renal failure

Other
  Bacteraemia or sepsis
  Multiorgan failure
  Psychological consequences
  Endocrine dysfunction
  Pressure sores

---

be improved by regular flexion and extension of the ankles or by calf compression with elastic stockings or inflatable cuffs. However, there is some doubt about the efficacy of these methods so most patients will require treatment with subcutaneous heparin or other anticoagulants.

A further problem is the prevention of gastrointestinal bleeding due to stress ulceration of the gastric mucosa. Stress ulceration is most common in patients who have suffered major trauma or severe haemorrhage and shock, and in those with sepsis, renal failure, and jaundice. Acute lung disease, especially ARDS, prolonged mechanical ventilation, and bleeding diatheses are additional risk factors. Three prophylactic regimens are commonly used: enteral nutrition, alkalis, and H_2 receptor blockers. Each regimen has advantages and disadvantages, and there is no general agreement as to which is most effective. Part of the difficulty is that the apparent incidence of ulceration depends on the method used to detect it. Whereas gastroscopy has revealed a high incidence of ulceration (75–100% in trauma patients) the incidence of bleeding observed at gastroscopy was less. The incidence of bleeding detected by occult blood was even smaller. Massive bleeding appears to occur in about 2–10% of a general population in the intensive care unit.

Enteral feeding has been shown to reduce the incidence of bleeding but may result in diarrhoea, tracheal and gastric colonisation, and nosocomial pneumonia. Alkalis have been found to be more effective in increasing gastric pH than cimetidine, but alkalis may cause diarrhoea, hypophosphataemia, hypomagnesia, and metabolic acidosis; H_2 blockers may cause renal failure and mental confusion, and cimetidine may produce drug interactions. A recent review of 16 studies comparing alkalis and cimetidine showed that both regimens were equally effective in preventing overt gastrointestinal bleeding.[39,41]

Another problem associated with the immobility of patients in the intensive care unit is skin necrosis. Regular changes of position and appropriate skin care are essential. If the patient is unconscious, care must be taken to tape the eyes shut after each instillation of antibiotic eye drops. Regular mouth care must be supplemented by movement of the tracheal tube and harness to ensure that pressure necrosis does not occur. The tracheal cuff may require reinflation at intervals to ensure that there is no leak around the cuff. The pressure should be checked by inserting a manometer into the inflation line and ensuring that the pressure is in the range of 20–25 cm H_2O.

Monitoring

Respiratory status. During spontaneous ventilation the best monitors are the respiratory rate, the pattern and depth of breathing, and the blood gases. The respiratory rate will obviously be affected by respiratory depressant drugs but is otherwise a sensitive indicator of the state of the patient's lungs. An increase in respiratory rate occurs during the development of pulmonary oedema and alveolar collapse and often signals the onset of an acute infection in patients with chronic lung disease. An increase in rate during weaning from mechanical ventilation usually indicates that muscle power is inadequate. A slowing of respiratory rate is one of the signs of opiate overdosage, but it may fail to provide an adequate warning of apnoea when the epidural route has been used.

The pattern of breathing provides a great deal of information to the skilled observer. Asynchronous movements of the abdomen and chest wall and activity in the accessory muscles of respiration suggest an increased work of breathing; a localised decrease in movement suggests underlying collapse, consolidation, or fluid. The estimation of tidal volume from observation of chest wall movements is subject to a high degree of error and should be checked with a portable spirometer. Similarly the degree of airway obstruc-

217

Monitoring of ventilation

Spontaneous
  Respiratory rate
  Pattern and depth of breathing
  Synchrony of abdominal and thoracic components
  Presence of accessory muscle activity
  Neural drive: $P_{0.1}$
  Inspiratory force
  Peak expiratory flow rate
  Vital capacity

Mechanical
  Inspired oxygen concentration
  Inspired temperature
  Expired volume
  Airway pressure profile
  Respiratory mechanics
  Intrinsic PEEP

Both
  Pulse oximetry
  Capnography
  Blood gases

tion in patients with airway obstruction should be measured with a peak flow meter.

In mechanically ventilated patients the airway pressure profile, the expired volume, and the oxygen concentration and temperature of inspired gas will usually be displayed continuously. Other ventilator variables such as I:E ratio, peak inspiratory flow rate, inspiratory flow pattern, or PEEP level may be displayed simultaneously or on demand. Many ventilators also provide information concerning compliance, resistance, intrinsic PEEP, and the patient's spontaneous respiratory activity. In general, the number of monitored variables increases with the complexity of the ventilator. There is much to be said for restricting the number of modes used so that both nurses and doctors can become familiar with the important variables that need to be monitored.

The use of a pulse oximeter is now routine, but it must be remembered that this provides a late warning of failure or disconnection of the oxygen supply if the patient has been receiving added oxygen. Pulse oximeters may give inaccurate readings when skin perfusion is reduced by arterial disease, cold, or shock or there is venous congestion. The readings may also be in error in patients with tricuspid incompetence. Although intravascular oxygen electrodes have proved useful in neonates they are subject to drift and have been little used in adult units. Transcutaneous electrodes for oxygen and carbon dioxide have proved relatively unreliable because the readings are greatly affected by variations in skin blood flow.

Most units now have a dedicated automated blood gas analyser, which eliminates most of the errors due to delay in analysis and to calibration of the electrodes. However, careless blood sampling can result in errors due to excessive volumes of heparin or the failure to maintain anaerobic conditions within the syringe by admitting air bubbles. Withdrawing the blood rapidly while the patient is hyperventilating or holding his or her breath can also result in important errors.

Cardiovascular monitoring. The use of a cardiac monitor and indirect or direct arterial pressure monitoring is routine. Central venous pressure monitoring is of value as a guide to transfusion when blood volume is reduced and is essential when rapid transfusion is required in an anaemic patient. The response to a rapid transfusion of 100–200 ml of fluid is of particular value for diagnosis in a patient with unexplained sudden hypotension that might be due, for example, to a pulmonary embolus or to concealed blood loss. The central venous pressure is also of value in controlling the right heart filling pressure in patients with cardiac failure.

It will be necessary to pass a flow directed pulmonary artery catheter if cardiac output measurements are required or if it becomes necessary to manipulate left atrial pressure to achieve an increased cardiac output. Care should be taken to ensure that the tip of the catheter is situated in a dependent zone of the lung, and measurements of pulmonary capillary wedge pressure should be made at the end of expiration and not during disconnection from the ventilator. Measurements of mixed venous saturation provide information on the relation between oxygen consumption and oxygen delivery and can be used to determine the appropriate dose levels when inotropes are being used to optimise oxygen delivery.

Other monitoring. Fluid intake, gastric aspirate, urine output, and the patient's temperature must be recorded at regular intervals. Scoring of coma level, depth of sedation, pain, and anxiety may also be required. If muscle relaxants are being used, it will be necessary to make regular checks of the degree of neuromuscular block with a nerve stimulator.

Weaning from respiratory support

Weaning difficulties are most common in patients who have received prolonged respiratory support or have suffered from some form of neuromuscular paralysis, and in those who have a history of chronic lung disease or a debilitating illness. The incidence of failure to wean within 24 hours of discontinuing support varies widely between units. It may be as low as 1–5% in patients who have been electively ventilated after cardiac surgery and as

---

Weaning

Difficulties
   Lack of central drive
   Abnormalities of neuromuscular system
   Increased respiratory load

Prerequisites
   Alert, cooperative patient
   Acute phase of disease process has finished
   Reasonable pattern and depth of spontaneous breathing between mandatory
      breaths
   Normal fluid balance and acid-base status

---

high as 20–30% in some other situations. However, most patients can be weaned within 5–7 days. Weaning difficulties may be due to a lack of central drive, abnormalities of the neuromuscular system, or an increased respiratory load. Often the causes are multifactorial.

Central drive

Central drive may be reduced by hypoxic, ischaemic, or direct damage to the respiratory centre. It may also be decreased by hyperventilation, a non-respiratory alkalosis, a reduction in hypoxic drive from the peripheral chemoreceptors, sleep loss, and drug depression. Most patients receive some form of sedation or analgesia during treatment. Normally, the short action of such drugs is due to redistribution, metabolism, or excretion. A drug such as thiopentone, which owes its short action to redistribution, will obviously accumulate when given repeatedly. It is therefore unsuitable for use in an intensive care unit. A drug such as morphine, which has active metabolites that are excreted through the kidney, may have a prolonged action in patients with renal failure. The long term effects produced by many drugs given in the intensive care unit are often underestimated by those who do not habitually work in this environment; these drugs should be the first factor to be considered when the patient fails to breathe.[42]

The neuromuscular system

A strong central drive may fail to generate an adequate response if there is an abnormality in the neuromuscular system. After a paralytic type of respiratory failure, recovery of muscle function may be slow and incomplete. There may be unsuspected weakness in patients with myasthenia gravis[43] and the prolonged administration of neuromuscular blocking agents often leads to cumulation and delayed recovery. Muscle contraction may be impaired by decreases in potassium,[44] calcium,[45] magnesium,[46] and phosphate ions.[47] Muscle power may also be reduced by disuse atrophy or by malnutrition.[48] There is some evidence that diaphragmatic function may be decreased by fatigue and that this may be accentuated by cardiogenic shock,[49] sepsis,[50] or an increased PCO_2.[51] Unilateral and bilateral diaphragmatic paralysis has been reported after open heart surgery, and diaphragm function is reduced after abdominal operations.[52] Thus there are many potential causes of respiratory muscle weakness at the time of weaning.

The respiratory load

It is a general policy to attempt weaning at the earliest possible time to minimise the complications associated with an artificial airway. Many of these patients will still have impaired lung function, so there will still be abnormalities of gas exchange and the respiratory muscles will have to work against an increased elastic or resistive load. It is usually the resistive component that creates the greatest problems. Part of the reason for this is that the respiratory muscles work inefficiently when the lungs are hyper-inflated. The minute volume is usually increased to cope with the increased ratio of dead space to tidal volume so that the work of breathing and the oxygen consumption are increased. This further increases the load.

In patients with a reduced compliance, FRC may be reduced when the respiratory support is withdrawn, and this may impair gas exchange and increase the work of breathing. In patients with borderline left ventricular failure, discontinuing respiratory support may precipitate failure and so cause pulmonary oedema. Another problem is that the patient still has to overcome the resistance of the tracheal tube, connections, and breathing system. This may easily double the work of breathing.

Techniques for weaning

Many attempts have been made to derive indices that predict successful weaning, but most have proved to be of little practical value (box). A better degree of prediction is usually obtained by measuring breathing frequency and tidal volume 5 minutes after disconnecting the patient from respiratory support.[53] The inspired oxygen concentration is maintained at the same level as that used during support, and the CPAP level is set to the PEEP level used on the ventilator. The normal ratio of frequency divided by tidal volume (in litres) is less than 30. A ratio of less than 80 suggests that patients may be weaned successfully, but few patients can be weaned if the ratio exceeds 105. The decision to start weaning is usually based on continued observation throughout the patient's stay in the unit. The patient should be alert and cooperative, should clearly be over the acute phase of the disease process,

---

Predictors for successful weaning

Tidal volume	>5 ml/kg
Vital capacity	>10-15 ml/kg
Respiratory rate	<30 bpm
Maximum inspiratory force	>-2.5 to -3.0 kPa (-25 to -30 cm H_2O)
PaO_2 (FIO_2 0.4-0.5)	>8 kPa (60 mm Hg)
pH	>7.3
$Qs/QT\%$	$<20\%$
VD/VT	<0.6

---

should be capable of generating a reasonable pattern and depth of spontaneous breathing between mandatory breaths, and should have a normal fluid balance and acid-base status. If the patient is being treated by bronchodilator drugs, a suitable dose should be given before starting weaning. The patient should be informed about the proposed weaning technique and should be warned that the process may take several days. It is important that the patient should have full confidence in the attendant who is to supervise the weaning, and it is better to return the patient to the support mode at the first sign of discomfort than to wait until respiratory distress develops.

Although there have been many studies of methods of weaning, no one technique has been shown to be better than any other. The simplest method is to disconnect the patient from the ventilator and to allow short periods of breathing from a high flow T piece system. The gas should contain a high concentration of oxygen to ensure that the patient does not become hypoxic, and it should be fully humidified. If the patient is likely to have a reduced compliance or has been receiving PEEP it is usually helpful to start weaning with a similar level of CPAP so that the tidal volume is situated on the steep part of the pressure-volume curve and the work of breathing is minimised. The periods of spontaneous breathing should initially be short (2–3 minutes) and should be extended as confidence is gained. In those who are likely to take several days to wean it is best to return the patient to full support at night in an attempt to secure a satisfactory period of sleep. Extubation should preferably be carried out in the morning and should be preceded by suction and a period of preoxygenation. Facilities for reintubation should be at hand and the patient observed closely for 12–24 hours after extubation because of the risk of laryngeal oedema or retention of secretions.

The other methods of weaning involve gradually reducing the frequency of mandatory breaths if the patient is on IMV or SIMV and reducing the level of pressure if the patient is on inspiratory pressure support. Again it may prove helpful to maintain the pre-existing PEEP level in the early stages of weaning. It has also been suggested that nasal intermittent positive pressure ventilation may prove helpful in particularly resistant cases (chapter 10).

Conclusions

The care of a patient in an intensive care unit now often involves the treatment of multiorgan failure. The assessment and monitoring of such patients provides complex problems for the clinician, and their day to day care creates a heavy burden for the nursing staff. Successful treatment can be achieved only by systematic consideration of the performance of each organ at frequent intervals and by using appropriate treatment. This entails keeping detailed records and ensuring that there are good communications between all grades of staff. It is important to remember that the patient and the relatives are at the centre of all this activity and that they should be kept informed of all aspects of treatment by senior members of the staff. The traditional ward round with discussion of the patient's condition at the foot of the bed is no longer tenable in intensive care, for the patient who is apparently deeply sedated may well overhear serious prognostications and thus suffer unnecessary anxiety.

1 Mascheroni D, Langer M, Marcolin M, Ronzoni G, Fumagalli R, Gattinoni L. Functional residual capacity is higher in CPAP than in CPPV with anaesthesia and in paralysis. *Intensive Care Med* 1986;**12**:228.

2 Katz JA, Marks JD. Inspiratory work with and without continuous positive airway pressure in patients with acute respiratory failure. *Anesthesiology* 1985;**63**:598–607.

3 Räsänen J, Väisänen IT, Heikkilä J, Nikki P. Acute myocardial infarction complicated by left ventilcular dysfunction and respiratory failure: the effects of continuous positive airway pressure. *Chest* 1985;**87**:158–62.

4 Duncan AW, Oh TE, Hillman DR. PEEP and CPAP. *Anaesth Intensive Care* 1986;**14**:236–50.

5 Gachot B, Clair B, Wolff M, Régnier B, Vachon F. Continuous airway pressure by facemask or mechanical ventilation in patients with human immunodeficiency virus infection and severe *Pneumocystis carinii* pneumonia. *Intensive Care Med* 1992;**18**:155–9.

6 Rotheram EB, Safar P, Robin E. CNS disorder during mechanical ventilation in chronic pulmonary disease. *JAMA* 1964;**189**:993–6.

7 Hickling KG, Henderson SJ, Jackson R. Low mortality associated with low volume pressure limited ventilation with permissive hypercapnia in severe adult respiratory distress syndrome. *Intensive Care Med* 1990;**16**:372–7.

8 Clark JM, Lambertson CJ. Pulmonary oxygen toxicity: a review. *Pharmacol Rev* 1971;**23**:37–133.

9 Suter PM, Fairley HB, Isenberg MD. Optimum end-expiratory pressure in patients with acute pulmonary failure. *N Engl J Med* 1975;**292**:284–9.

10 Tenaillon A, Labrousse J, Gateau O, Lissac J. Optimum positive end-expiratory pressure and static lung compliance. *N Engl J Med* 1978;**299**:774–5.

11 Murray IP, Modell JH, Gallagher TJ, Banner MJ. Titration of PEEP by the arterial minus end-tidal carbon dioxide gradient. *Chest* 1984;**85**:100–4.

12 Jardin F, Genevray B, Pazin M, Margairaz A. Inability to titrate PEEP in patients with acute respiratory failure using end-tidal carbon dioxide measurements. *Anesthesiology* 1985;**62**:530–3.

13 Matamis D, Lemaire F, Harf A, Brun-Buisson C, Ansquer JC, Atlan G. Total respiratory pressure–volume curves in the adult respiratory distress syndrome. *Chest* 1984;**86**:58–66.

14 Kirby RR, Downs JB, Civetta JM, Modell JH, Dannemiller FJ, Klein EF, *et al.* High level positive end expiratory pressure (PEEP) in acute respiratory insufficiency. *Chest* 1975;**67**:156–65.

15 Jardin F, Desfond P, Bazin M, Sportiche M, Margairez A. Controlled ventilation with best

positive end-expiratory pressure (PEEP) and a high level PEEP in acute respiratory failure (ARF). *Intensive Care Med* 1981;**7**:171–6.

16 Pepe PE, Hudson LD, Carrico CJ. Early application of positive end-expiratory pressure in patients at risk for the adult respiratory distress syndrome. *N Engl J Med* 1984;**311**:281–6.

17 Carroll GC, Tuman KJ, Braverman B, Logas WG, Wool N, Goldin M, *et al.* Minimal positive end-expiratory pressure (PEEP) may be "best PEEP." *Chest* 1988;**93**:1020–5.

18 Eissa NT, Ranieri VM, Corbell C, Chassé M, Braidy J, Robatto FM, *et al.* Analysis of behavior of the respiratory system in ARDS patients: effects of flow, volume, and time. *J Appl Physiol* 1991;**70**:2719–29.

19 Ranieri VM, Eissa NT, Corbell C, Chassé M, Braidy M, Matar N, *et al.* Effects of positive end-expiratory pressure on alveolar recruitment and gas exchange in patients with the adult respiratory distress syndrome. *Am Rev Respir Dis* 1991;**144**:544–51.

20 Dall'Ava-Santucci J, Armaganidis A, Brunet F, Dhainhaut J-F, Nouira S, Morisseau D, *et al.* Mechanical effects of PEEP in patients with adult respiratory distress syndrome. *J Appl Physiol* 1991;**68**:843–8.

21 Braun NMT, Faulkner J, Hughes RL, Roussos C, Sahgal V. When should respiratory muscles be exercised? *Chest* 1983;**84**:76–84.

22 Brochard L. Inspiratory pressure support. *Eur J Anaesthesiol* 1994;**11**:29–36.

23 Wahba RWM. Pressure support ventilation. *J Cardiothoracic Anesth* 1990;**4**:624–30.

24 Tokioka H, Saito S, Kosaka F. Effect of pressure support on breathing patterns and respiratory work. *Intensive Care Med* 1989;**15**:491–4.

25 Falkenhain S, Reilly T, Gregory J. Improvement in cardiac output during airway pressure release ventilation. *Crit Care Med* 1992;**20**:1358–60.

26 Valentine DD, Hammond MD, Downs JB, Sears NJ, Sims WR. Distribution of ventilation and perfusion with different modes of mechanical ventilation. *Am Rev Respir Dis* 1991;**143**:1262–6.

27 Osborne RJ, Joel JP, Slevin ML. Morphine intoxication in rental failure: the role of morphine-6-glucuronide. *BMJ* 1986;**292**:1548–9.

28 Shelly MP, Quinn KG, Park GR. Pharmacokinetics of morphine in patients following orthoptic liver transplantation. *Br J Anaesth* 1989;**63**:375–9.

29 Sinclair MER, Sear JW, Summerfield RJ, Fisher A. Alfentanil infusions on the intensive care unit. *Intensive Care Med* 1988;**14**:55–9.

30 Scott DB, Beamish D, Hudson IN, Jostell K-G. Prolonged infusion of chlormethiazole in intensive care. *Br J Anaesth* 1980;**52**:541–5.

31 Spencer EM, Willatts SM. Isoflurane infusion for prolonged sedation in the intensive care unit: efficacy and safety. *Intensive Care Med* 1992;**18**:415–21.

32 Truog RD, Rice SA. Inorganic fluoride and prolonged isoflurane anesthesia in the intensive care unit. *Anesth Analg* 1989;**69**:843–5.

33 Isenstein DA, Venner DS, Duggan J. Neuromuscular blockade in the intensive care unit. *Chest* 1992;**102**:1258–66.

34 Parker CJR, Jones JE, Hunter JM. Disposition of infusions of atracurium and its metabolite, laudanosine, in patients in renal and respiratory failure in an ITU. *Br J Anaesth* 1988;**61**:531–40.

35 Christman JW, McCain RW. A sensible approach to the nutritional support of mechanically ventilated critically ill patients. *Intensive Care Med* 1993;**19**:129–36.

36 Braun U, Zundel J, Freiboth K, Weyland W, Turner E, Heidelmeyer CF, *et al.* Evaluation of methods for indirect calorimetry with a ventilated lung model. *Intensive Care Med* 1989;**15**:196–202.

37 Merilainen PT. Metabolic monitor. *Int J Clin Monit Comput* 1987;**4**:167–77.

38 Zwillich CW, Pierson DJ, Creagh CE, Sutton FD, Schatz E, Petty TL. Complications of assisted ventilation. A prospective study of 354 consecutive episodes. *Am J Med* 1974;**57**:161–70.

39 Pingleton SK. Complications of acute respiratory failure. *Am Rev Respir Dis* 1988;**137**:1463–93.

40 Symposium on nosocomial infection and use of selective decontamination. *Intensive Care Med* 1992;**18**:S1–38.

41 Noseworthy TW, Cook DJ. Noscomial pneumonia, prophylaxis against gastric erosive

disease, and clinically important gastric bleeding: where do we stand? *Crit Care Med* 1993;**21**: 1814–6.
42 Sear JW. Overview of drugs available for ITU sedation. *Eur J Anaesthesiol* 1987;**1**(suppl): 47–53.
43 Mier-Jedrzezowicz A, Brophy C, Green M. Respiratory muscle function in myasthenia gravis. *Am Rev Respir Dis* 1988;**138**:867–73.
44 Knockel JP. Neuromuscular manifestations of electrolyte disorders. *Am J Med* 1982;**72**: 521–35.
45 Aubier M, Viires N, Piquet J, Murciano D, Blanchet F, Marty C, *et al.* Effects of hypocalcaemia on diaphragmatic strength generation. *J Appl Physiol* 1985;**58**:2054–61.
46 Dhingra S, Solven F, Wilson A, McCarthy DS. Hypomagnesemia and respiratory muscle power. *Am Rev Respir Dis* 1984;**129**:497–8.
47 Aubier M, Murciano D, Lecocguic Y, Viires N, Jacquens Y, Squara P, *et al.* Effect of hypophosphatemia on diaphragmatic contractility in patients with acute respiratory failure. *N Engl J Med* 1985;**313**:420–4.
48 Larca L, Greenbaum DM. Effectiveness of intensive nutritional regimes in patients who fail to wean from mechanical ventilator. *Crit Care Med* 1982;**10**:297–300.
49 Aubier M, Trippenbach T, Roussos C. Respiratory muscle fatigue during cardiogenic shock. *J Appl Physiol* 1981;**51**:499–508.
50 Hussain SNA, Simkus G, Roussos C. Respiratory muscle fatigue: a cause of ventilatory failure in septic shock. *J Appl Physiol* 1985;**58**:2033–40.
51 Juan G, Galverley P, Talamo C, Schnader J, Roussos C. Effect of carbon dioxide on diaphragmatic function in human beings. *N Engl J Med* 1984;**310**:874–9.
52 Ford GT, Whitelaw WA, Rosenal TW, Cruse PJ, Guenter CA. Diaphragm function after upper abdominal surgery in humans. *Am Rev Respir Dis* 1983;**127**:431–6.
53 Goldstone J, Moxham J. Weaning from mechanical ventilation. In: Moxham J, Goldstone J, eds. *Assisted ventilation.* 2nd ed. London: BMJ Publications, 1994.

10 Non-invasive techniques of respiratory support

Previous chapters have dealt with techniques of respiratory support that require tracheal intubation or tracheostomy. This chapter describes methods of providing respiratory support without an artificial airway. These may be broadly divided into the "negative" pressure techniques, which produce an inspiration by generating a subatmospheric pressure around the chest wall, and the positive pressure techniques, which use a full face or nasal mask to connect a continuous or intermittent positive source to the lungs.

Although the former technique should strictly be termed "subatmospheric" pressure ventilation, this term is little used in the clinical environment, so the more commonly used term negative pressure ventilation has been retained throughout this chapter.

For many years the only non-invasive methods of assisting ventilation were the tank and cuirass ventilators. These were used mainly to maintain adequate ventilation in patients with poliomyelitis. In the 1980s two new developments created a renewed interest in non-invasive techniques. One was the recognition that the nocturnal use of non-invasive ventilatory assistance could reverse the blood gas changes and daytime respiratory symptoms in patients with certain forms of chronic respiratory failure.[1] The second was the recognition that the close fitting nasal masks designed for the delivery of continuous nasal positive airway pressure for the treatment of obstructive sleep apnoea[2] could also be used to deliver an intermittent positive pressure to the lungs. This development opened up exciting new possibilities for the use of these techniques in respiratory care.

Negative non-invasive techniques are now used mainly to provide long term support for patients with limited respiratory reserve and nocturnal hypoventilation due to restrictive disorders such as kyphoscoliosis, thoracoplasty, and residual paralysis from poliomyelitis. They are also useful when such patients develop acute respiratory infections, but they are of doubtful value in acute exacerbations of chronic obstructive airways disease.

Positive pressure techniques can provide effective support in patients with chronic respiratory failure due to restrictive conditions and seem to improve blood gases in acute exacerbations of chronic obstructive airways disease. They are also used to provide support pending lung transplantation, to facilitate weaning from conventional ventilation, and, occasionally, to improve cardiorespiratory status before surgery. There is an increasing

226

Prerequisites for successful non-invasive support

- Patient's cooperation
- Patient can control airway and secretions
- Adequate cough reflex
- Patient can breathe unaided for several minutes
- Functioning gastrointestinal tract
- Haemodynamic stability

---

recognition that positive pressure techniques can be used successfully to augment ventilation in many types of acute respiratory failure, and they are now widely used for treating central and obstructive sleep apnoea.

There are some essential prerequisites for successful non-invasive support. Patients must be cooperative, be able to control their own airway and secretions, and have an adequate cough reflex. As the mask may become displaced they must be able to breathe on their own for several minutes. They should also have a functioning gastrointestinal tract and be haemodynamically stable.

For convenience the non-invasive methods will be divided into intermittent negative pressure and intermittent positive pressure techniques. The choice of method depends partly on the condition being treated but is also governed by the patient's wishes and the local availability of expertise and equipment.

Intermittent negative pressure ventilation

The term intermittent negative pressure ventilation is used to denote a method of producing lung expansion by intermittently reducing the absolute pressure around the chest wall. The only negative pressure device capable of providing long term total respiratory support in patients with abnormalities of the lungs or chest wall is the tank ventilator or "iron lung." Cuirass or jacket ventilators also produce lung inflation by creating a subatmospheric pressure around the chest wall, but their efficiency is reduced by air leaks and they are usually only capable of providing partial support.

Tank ventilators

A tank ventilator consists of a large, rigid container which surrounds the whole of the patient's body except the head and neck. An airtight seal around the neck is produced by a rubber collar and the pressure inside the tank is intermittently lowered below atmospheric by a large, mechanically driven bellows or high capacity rotary pump. A tank ventilator can provide adequate

Methods of producing INPV

Tank ventilators
   Laryngeal function is preserved
   Not suitable for patients with severe acute lung disease
   Expensive
   Need much space
   Discomfort from neck seal and immobility
   Medical and nursing procedures difficult

Cuirass ventilators
   Problems due to leaks now reduced by tailored shells and better pumps
   Sleeping position restricted
   Pressure sores may develop

Jacket ventilators
   Do not restrict chest movement
   Fewer problems with pressure sores
   Air leaks
   Back board may be uncomfortable

ventilation in patients who have normal swallowing mechanisms and moderately impaired lung function, but it cannot generate sufficiently high subatmospheric pressures to treat patients with severe acute lung disease. The great advantage of the method is that laryngeal function is preserved, so that the patient can speak, and the complications associated with a tracheostomy are avoided. However, tank ventilators are expensive, they require a large floor area (to enable the patient to be slid in and out of the machine), and the patient suffers discomfort from the neck seal and from the immobility enforced by the supine position. There are also difficulties in carrying out medical and nursing procedures through the portholes in the walls of the machine. Patients with almost complete paralysis will require nursing in the tank ventilator for the whole 24 hours, but those with some respiratory muscle activity can often be removed from the tank and assisted by some other device during the day. Under these circumstances the possibility of preserving laryngeal function by the use of a tank ventilator may offset its disadvantages.

The simple Both design of tank ventilator was in widespread use in the United Kingdom until the 1950s but was then superseded by a series of new machines designed by Smith-Clarke (a retired motor company engineer) and manufactured by the Cape Engineering Company in Warwick.[3] In the improved machines the upper half of the headboard sloped away from the patient, so that tracheostomy care was facilitated if this became necessary, and a mirror could be provided to extend the patient's range of view. The tank was split horizontally and hinged at the foot end so that it could be

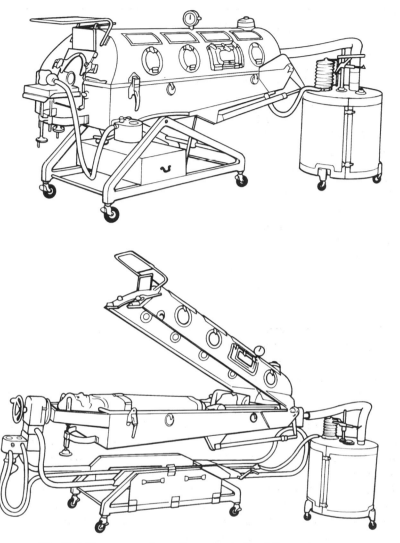

Fig 10.1 Coventry tank ventilator: (top) closed (bottom) open.

opened like an alligator's jaws (fig 10.1). Multiple ports were provided for intravenous infusions and nursing care, and in the most sophisticated machines the patient could be tilted or rotated through 180° to facilitate physiotherapy and skin care.[4]

In recent years a more portable, polycarbonate tank ventilator, the Lifecare Portalung, has been developed. This is available in three sizes and uses a large displacement rotary pump, rather than a bellows to evacuate the chamber during each inspiration. Inflation pressures of -15 to -35 cm H_2O

229

are required to generate normal tidal volumes in patients with relatively normal lungs. It must be remembered that these pressures are applied to the whole trunk and so depress the cardiovascular system in a similar manner to positive pressure applied to the airway (see chapter 2).

Tank ventilators are now found only in special units that cater for patients with chronic neuromuscular paralysis. They are used to maintain ventilation in patients who have normal pharyngeal and laryngeal function and so do not require a tracheostomy. Patients with partial paralysis may be able to maintain adequate ventilation with a cuirass, rocking bed, or abdominal belt during the day but may require treatment with a tank at night. Tank ventilators are often used to provide temporary support for patients with limited respiratory reserve when they develop a respiratory infection. Nocturnal support by tank ventilator has also been used to improve the blood gases in patients with chronic lung disease, but the value of this type of treatment is difficult to assess.[5]

Cuirass and jacket ventilators

From the circulatory point of view the ideal method of ventilating the lungs is to apply intermittent subatmospheric pressure to the chest wall, for this generates the same gradient of pressure between the peripheral and central veins, as does a spontaneous inspiration. Unfortunately, the difficulty in achieving a satisfactory seal between the device and the chest wall has limited the application of the technique.

The earliest attempts to produce ventilation by this method used a rigid shell applied to the front of the thorax. The first such device was introduced by Eisenmenger in 1904, the negative pressure being generated by the expansion of a spring loaded, foot operated bellows. In 1927 he patented a mechanical version of this device (the Biomotor), which applied both positive and subatmospheric pressure to the front of the chest and abdomen.[6] A similar device was developed by Sahlin in Sweden and used to treat 827 patients with poliomyelitis, of whom 127 survived.[7] During the 1930s the Burstall jacket in Australia and the London County Council cuirass in Britain were widely used to treat respiratory paralysis due to poliomyelitis, but there were always difficulties in achieving an airtight seal with the limited range of shells available.[6]

In the 1960s a number of anaesthetists attempted to use cuirass ventilators to maintain ventilation when the patient was anaesthetised and paralysed to permit the passage of a rigid bronchoscope. It was soon found that it was difficult to achieve adequate ventilation in obese patients and in those with chronic lung disease or abnormally shaped chests.[8]

The Tunnicliffe jacket was introduced in an attempt to solve these problems. This consisted of a cotton-nylon jacket that was sealed by straps across the arms, neck, and buttocks but held away from the chest by a plastic frame. This proved reasonably efficient, but the relatively large air leak often made the patient feel cold.[9] J H Emerson produced a similar design in the United States.[10]

Modern jackets resemble an anorak with hood and enclose the head, neck, and arms. This improves the seal but prevents their use in the patient with a tracheostomy. The jackets are sealed by elasticated cuffs around the limbs and abdomen, but some also enclose the thighs in an attempt to minimise the air leak into the interior. This design may decrease patient mobility and increase the difficulties of nursing care. The jackets are manufactured in two sizes and should fit patients of widely differing sizes and shapes, but the larger may be too small for some patients with scoliosis. The jacket is held away from the chest by a frame and does not restrict chest movement, so it may be more efficient than the cuirass in some patients. It also minimises problems with pressure sores. However, the plastic frame which surrounds the chest is mounted on a back board and this may create discomfort.

During the past two decades there has been a resurgence of interest in the use of cuirass ventilators. This is due to improvements in the design of the shell and pump. The shape of the shell can now be matched to each patient by taking a plaster cast of the patient's thorax and using this as a mould to construct the shell from fibreglass or other lightweight material. The shell extends from the manubrium to the lower abdomen and makes contact with the chest wall as far back as possible so that the seal is augmented by contact of the shell with the mattress. By padding the edges with foam rubber and covering them with an airtight material such as neoprene, a shell that is both light and airtight can be constructed at reasonable cost.[11] The shell may then be held in contact with the thorax by a wide strap which passes round the trunk.

The efficiency of the cuirass has been further improved by replacing the large bellows units which generated the subatmospheric pressure by specially designed rotary pumps. These have a high flow capability so that they can achieve a predetermined subatmospheric pressure despite small leaks.[12] Since tidal volume is linearly related to the subatmospheric pressure,[13] this ensures that ventilation is reasonably well maintained as long as there is no gross leak. The disadvantages of the cuirass are that the patient has to sleep on the back or slightly inclined to one side, and that pressure sores may develop where the shell presses on the skin. Most cuirass devices provide controlled ventilation, but a patient triggered model is available.

Indications for negative pressure ventilation

Cuirass ventilators are most often used to augment ventilation in patients with chronic respiratory inadequancy of neuromuscular or skeletal origin; their regular use results in an improvement in blood gases during both the day and night.[13] If the underlying disease is not progressive the long term prognosis is also improved.[14] In some patients treated by cuirass the ventilation can be maintained at an adequate level throughout the 24 hours, but other patients may need to sleep in a tank ventilator at night.

The cuirass is also useful when patients with chronic neuromuscular disease or skeletal deformities develop acute respiratory infections.[15] In patients with a severe limitation of lung function it may be necessary to use a tank ventilator for the first few days of treatment, but in others a tank may only be required to avoid the inevitable respiratory depression associated with sleep.

A controversial use for negative pressure ventilation has been in the long term treatment of chronic obstructive airways disease, the theory being that providing nocturnal assistance to ventilation might rest the respiratory muscles and so decrease fatigue. Recent studies have shown that regular negative pressure ventilation in a tank can increase respiratory muscle strength and endurance,[16,17] but whether this improves the quality of life or survival is not clear.[18-20] Negative pressure ventilation has also been advocated for treating the sleep apnoea syndrome. It may prove useful in patients with episodes of apnoea of central origin, but it is of little value in those with obstructive apnoea—sleep abolishes the normal pharyngeal mechanisms that hold the airway open during inspiration, and the subatmospheric airway pressure generated by the negative pressure ventilator accentuates the airway obstruction.[21] Nocturnal airway obstruction is one of the major drawbacks to any negative pressure technique.

Other devices acting on the chest wall

Rocking bed

Another method of providing partial ventilatory support is the rocking bed (fig 10.2). This is based on the Eve method of artificial ventilation.[22] The patient reclines in a semirecumbent position on a special bed that permits the patient to be rocked between a head up and head down position at respiratory frequencies. The variation in pressure exerted by the abdominal contents on the diaphragm augments the spontaneous diaphragmatic activity and permits patients with limited respiratory activity to spend several hours out of the tank ventilator. The bed is usually fitted with a face mask attachment that can

---

Devices that act on the chest wall

- Rocking bed
- Diaphragmatic pacing
- High frequency chest wall oscillation
- Intermittent abdominal compression

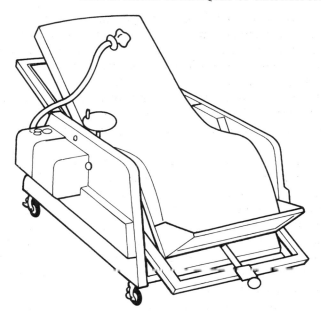

Fig 10.2 Rocking bed. Bed can be rocked through an angle of about 40° at respiratory frequencies.

deliver an intermittent positive pressure supply of air. This is synchronised with the movements of the bed and enables the patient to augment the tidal volume when required. Not surprisingly, a proportion of patients are unable to use the bed because of nausea and vomiting. For others, however, it provides a welcome respite from the discomfort of the tank.[21] Some patients can also learn to augment the ventilation by using the pharyngeal muscles to force gulps of air into the lungs—a technique known as glossopharyngeal breathing.

Diaphragmatic pacing

Electrical stimulation of the phrenic nerve to maintain ventilation for long periods was first reported in 1968 and has now been used in several hundred patients, some of whom have been treated for 10–15 years.[24] It can be used only in those who have an intact lower motor neurone with normal diaphragmatic muscle. It has therefore been used mainly in patients with the primary alveolar hypoventilation syndrome[25] and in those with quadriplegia due to to a lesion above the third cervical segment.[26] An external, battery powered transmitter generates a radiofrequency signal which is radiated from a loop antenna. The antenna is placed over a subcutaneous receiver, which is encapsulated in an epoxy resin disc and covered with silicone rubber. The

233

receiver demodulates the signal and generates direct current pulses, which are fed to electrodes placed on each phrenic nerve (usually in the neck). The duration and frequency of inspiration can be controlled by the timing of the train of stimuli and the tidal volume can be controlled by the intensity of the stimulus. To avoid diaphragm fatigue and irreversible damage to the muscle, each diaphragm is paced in turn for a period of up to 16 hours.

High frequency chest wall oscillation

High frequency oscillation applied to the chest wall of apnoeic animals has been shown to increase carbon dioxide elimination, but attempts to use this technique in humans by applying oscillations to a cuff surrounding the chest resulted in a reduction in functional residual capacity. To overcome this problem a new device, the Hayek oscillator, has been developed. This consists of a cuirass, which surrounds the chest, connected to a power source capable of maintaining a standing subatmospheric pressure with superimposed oscillations. A recent trial of this device in patients with severe chronic obstructive airways disease using oscillating pressures of -10 to -26 cm H_2O at frequencies ranging from 60 to 140 breaths/min showed a reduction in PCO_2 and increases in arterial saturation in both normocapnic and hypercapnic patients.[27] This device may prove useful in the provision of temporary support in other types of ventilatory failure.

Intermittent abdominal compression

The first device using this principle was the Bragg–Paul pulsator.[28] This consisted of a pneumatic band placed around the lower chest and intermittently inflated, inspiration occurring when the band was deflated. This was unable to generate adequate tidal volumes and had the additional disadvantage that it compressed the chest and so encouraged atelectasis. Although the method was recently resuscitated, using an abdominal belt to treat patients with respiratory insufficiency due to a neuromuscular disease, it was successful in only about half of the patients treated.[29]

Positive pressure techniques

Continuous positive airway pressure breathing (CPAP)

There are two main indications for the use of continuous positive pressure breathing. The first is its use with a face mask to prevent alveolar collapse during expiration in patients with pulmonary oedema, pneumonia, or ARDS, so minimising the intrapulmonary shunt and improving arterial oxygenation. It has also been used for this purpose in those being weaned from mechanical ventilation. The second, and more recent, application is the use of a nasal CPAP to provide a pneumatic splint which holds the upper airway open in patients with nocturnal hypoxaemia due to episodes of obstructive sleep apnoea.

The basic principles of CPAP have already been discussed (pp 83–94). It was emphasised that there are three essential requirements for successful treatment. Firstly, the breathing system must not permit rebreathing. Secondly, the pressure during inspiration and expiration should not vary by more than 1–2 cm H_2O in order to minimise the work of breathing. Thirdly, the valve generating the positive pressure should have the characteristics of a threshold resistor so that the pressure in the system remains at the set levels despite variations in expiratory flow rate. Thus the breathing system and devices for generating the positive pressure are similar to those used in the intubated patient. However, the reduction in airway resistance resulting from the elimination of the tracheal tube and connections should reduce the variations in pressure within the airway.

CPAP may be administered by a closely fitting nasal or face mask. Masks are usually made from a non-irritant material such as silicone rubber and should have minimal dead space and a soft inflatable cuff to provide a seal with the skin. They should be held in place with a comfortable head harness. Particular care is necessary to ensure that the mask does not press on the bridge of the nose, as the skin in this area ulcerates quickly if pressure is excessive.

A full face mask is used when CPAP is being used to increase the functional residual capacity in patients with alveolar collapse. It is also commonly used in patients with acute exacerbations of chronic lung disease and in children, since such patients often breathe through the mouth. Pressures are usually limited to 5–10 cm H_2O, since higher pressures tend to result in gastric distension, which can be relieved only by continual aspiration through a nasogastric tube. In babies, who are habitual nose breathers, nasal prongs may be substituted for the mask. Nasal pillows or other nasal seals are available for patients who find a mask claustophobic or who develop skin necrosis from the mask.

In patients with obstructive sleep apnoea, upper airway patency is maintained by applying CPAP through a nasal mask, the pressure level being adjusted by direct observation during sleep.[2] Usually, considerable benefit is produced by pressure of 5–10 cm H_2O. Daytime symptoms disappear immediately, and there is a reduction in morbidity and mortality.[30] Some patients complain of nasal symptoms, however, and others find the mask claustrophobic, so compliance rates are usually about 60–75%. As the hypoxaemia is usually abolished by relief of the obstruction, the positive pressure can be produced by fairly simple devices that compress ambient air (fig 10.3, for example). More sophisticated devices are now available: these are patient cycled and alternate the pressure at respiratory frequencies, so augmenting CO_2 clearance as well.[31]

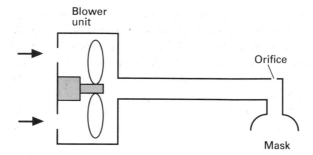

Fig 10.3 Simple CPAP device. Speed of rotation of fan in blower unit controls pressure in system. Expired gas initially passes back into tube but is then expelled through orifice (which is about 2 mm in diameter) during expiratory pause. CPAP pressure remains reasonably constant because efficiency of fan increases during inspiration and decreases during expiration in response to slight changes in pressure within mask.

Intermittent positive pressure ventilation

Many patients requiring respiratory support of limited duration can be treated effectively with IPPV given through a nasal mask or full face mask, or occasionally by a mouthpiece.[32] The technique is particularly useful in patients who require ventilation only at night—it eliminates the complications associated with intubation and the need for humidification and allows full mobility during the daytime.[33]

The main indications for the use of this technique are chronic respiratory failure due to thoracic deformity, the after effects of operative pulmonary ablation for the treatment of tuberculosis, or residual weakness from poliomyelitis or other slowly progressive neuromuscular disease.[34-37] These conditions tend to result in noctural hypoventilation and the later development of pulmonary hypertension and cor pulmonale, the onset of which can be delayed by the regular use of IPPV. In such patients an apparently trivial disturbance such as a minor respiratory infection or the administration of a sedative or a general anaesthetic can result in cardiorespiratory arrest and later difficulties in weaning from the ventilator in the intensive care unit. Patients with episodes of sleep apnoea due to central depression or airway obstruction may also benefit from this form of treatment.[38]

In recent years non-invasive positive pressure ventilation has been used increasingly to treat episodes of acute respiratory failure and of acute-on-chronic failure. It has recently been reported that intubation can be avoided in 50–75% of patients with acute respiratory failure[39, 40] and that survival is improved in patients with acute exacerbations of chronic obstructive airways disease.[41,42] Nasal ventilation has also been used to wean patients with chronic respiratory insufficiency from a ventilator.[43]

The successful use of a positive pressure system depends on the patient's

236

cooperation and this can be secured only if the patient is given detailed instructions. The patient should first be allowed to hold the mask on the face while small breaths are delivered. After a few minutes the size of the breath can be increased and the mask finally secured when the patient relaxes and coordinates the spontaneous breathing with the rhythm of the machine. Synchronisation with a controlled pattern of breathing is most easily accomplished in patients who are breathless or drifting off to sleep; it is often difficult to achieve effective synchronisation is those with a strong respiratory drive.

In patients with chronic obstructive airways disease and a chronically increased PCO_2 a small flow of oxygen (about 1 l/min) results in an increase in PCO_2 even if the ventilator is set appropriately. In such patients it is probably wise to check the blood gases after about 30 minutes' treatment. In other patients, monitoring by pulse oximeter and end tidal PCO_2 can provide a useful guide to the effectiveness of the treatment.

One of the major problems in patients being ventilated by a nasal mask is a leak through the mouth. The mouth can be held closed by an elasticated chin strap; if this is not effective a pressure generator can be used to provide better compensation for leaks. Patients may suffer from gastric distension, dryness or excessive mucus secretion in the nose, and the occasional epistaxis. Humidification is usually not required, but if secretions are viscid a heat and moisture exchanger or hot water humidifer may be inserted into the breathing system.

As the minute volume delivered by the ventilator must be one and a half times to twice the patient's minute volume to compensate for the increased dead space and the loss of gas through leaks around the mask, some conventional ventilators may prove inadequate. Several ventilators are specifically designed for home ventilation (see appendix). These may be flow or pressure generators but are usually time cycled from inspiration to expiration. Some have facilities for patient triggering, but the use of this mode is rendered more difficult by the frequency of leaks and movements of the patient. As some of these patients have apnoeic attacks while asleep, it is advisable to use a mode such as SIMV, which provides a mandatory breath if the patient does not trigger the ventilator within a preset time.

Recently there has been some interest in the use of patient cycled, biphasic positive airway pressure (BiPAP in the American literature) as a method of providing non-invasive ventilation by nasal mask. This differs from the BIPAP technique described in chapter 5 in that the BiPAP machine is cycled between the high and low pressures at respiratory frequencies in synchrony with the patient's spontaneous respiratory activity. It thus acts as a patient cycled pressure generator that provides inspiratory pressure support with PEEP. The Respironics BiPAP device is cycled from the low to the high pressure by an inspiratory flow of more than 40 ml/sec for more than 30 msec. Cycling from the high pressure to the low is initiated by a decrease in inspiratory flow below a threshold level, an increase in pressure above the preset level, or an inspiratory period exceeding 3 seconds. Similar machines are now available in Britain.

BiPAP machines have the advantage that they are pressure generators and so compensate for small leaks, but they do not incorporate the usual high and low pressure and disconnection alarms found on standard ventilators, so other forms of monitoring are required to ensure patient safety. The adjustment of the controls on this type of machine depends on the type of respiratory failure. In general the increase in pressure from the low to the high level effectively provides inspiratory pressure support and thus augments CO_2 elimination, while the lower level maintains end expiratory lung volume. The machine is initially set to cycle between 5 and 10 cm H_2O, the lower pressure being increased if there is unacceptable hypoxaemia and the difference between the two pressures being increased if increased CO_2 elimination is required. In one study, such a regimen resulted in the avoidance of intubation in approximately 75% of episodes of acute respiratory failure.[39]

This technique is worth trying in patients with mild or moderate ventilatory failure, but it must be remembered that it is inherently less safe than conventional forms of support. The lack of ventilator alarms increases the risk of an undetected hypoventilation or apnoea, so the technique should only be used when close and continued observation by trained staff can be provided.

Conclusions

The increased use of non-invasive methods of respiratory support has resulted in a reduction in the need for intubation or tracheostomy. This has had three major effects. Firstly, it has encouraged the use of assisted ventilation in the home.[44] Secondly, it has reduced the incidence of complications normally associated with the use of an artificial airway and shortened the average duration of treatment in the intensive care unit. Thirdly, it has eliminated some of the ethical dilemmas previously faced by doctors who were asked to treat respiratory failure in progressively debilitating conditions.[45]

There are still circumstances in which the initiation of respiratory support may not prolong life significantly, and in which it may ultimately cause increased distress to the patient or relatives. In such situations there is still a need for careful assessment and a full and frank discussion of the possible advantages and disadvantages with both the patient and relatives before non-invasive ventilation is started. However, the prognosis of many diseases is changing rapidly. For example, lung transplantation for terminal cystic fibrosis is now feasible, and nasal IPPV may be used successfully to stabilise patients awaiting a transplant.[46] Such changing perspectives provide a continual challenge to those engaged in providing respiratory support.

1 Garay SM, Turino GM, Goldring RM. Sustained reversal of chronic hypercapnia in patients with alveolar hypoventilation syndromes: long-term maintenance with noninvasive mechanical ventilation. *Am J Med* 1981;70:269–74.
2 Sullivan CE, Berthon-Jones M, Issa FG, Eves L. Reversal of obstructive sleep apnoea by continuous airway pressure applied through the nares. *Lancet* 1981;i:862–5.
3 Galpine JF. A new cabinet respirator. *Lancet* 1954;i:707–9.
4 Kelleher WH. A new pattern of "iron lung" for the prevention and treatment of airway complications in paralytic disease. *Lancet* 1961;ii:1113–6.
5 Hill NS. Non-invasive ventilation. Does it work, for whom, and how? *Am Rev Respir Dis* 1993;147:1050–5.
6 Woollam CHM. The development of apparatus for intermittent negative pressure respiration. 1919–1976, with special reference to the development and uses of cuirass respirators. *Anaesthesia* 1976;31:666–85.
7 Bergman R. Eight hundred cases of poliomyelitis treated in the Sahlin respirator. *Acta Paediatr* 1948;36:470.
8 Wallace G, Webb FI, Becker WH, Coppolino CA. The value of the cuirass respirator during anesthesia for endoscopy. *Anesth Analg* 1961;40:505–8.
9 Spalding JMK, Opie L. Artificial respiration with the Tunnicliffe breathing-jacket. *Lancet* 1958;i:613–5.
10 Halperin SW, Waskow WH. Emerson wrap-around chest respirator, for use in bronchoscopy and laryngoscopy. *Anesth Analg* 1959;38:440–50.
11 Brown L, Kinnear W, Sargeant K-A, Schneerson JM. Artificial ventilation by external negative pressure—a method of manufacturing cuirass shells. *Physiotherapy* 1985;71:181–3.
12 Kinnear WJM, Schneerson JM. The Newmarket pump: a new suction pump for negative pressure ventilation. *Thorax* 1985;40:677–81.
13 Kinnear W, Petch M, Taylor G, Schneerson JM. Assisted ventilation using cuirass ventilators. *Eur Respir J* 1988;1:198–203.
14 Edwards PR, Howard P. Methods and prognosis of non-invasive ventilation in neuromuscular disease. *Arch Chest Dis* 1993;48:176–82.
15 Libby DM, Briscoe WA, Boyce B, Smith JP. Acute respiratory failure in scoliosis and kyphosis. Prolonged survival and treatment. *Am J Med* 1982;73:532–8.
16 Scano G, Gigliotti F, Duranti R, Spinelli A, Gorini M, Schiavina M. Changes in ventilatory muscle function with negative pressure ventilation in patients with severe COPD. *Chest* 1990;97:322–7.
17 Cropp A, Dimarco AF. Effect of intermittent negative pressure ventilation on respiratory muscle function in patients with severe chronic obstructive pulmonary disease. *Am Rev Respir Dis* 1987;135:1056–61.
18 Zibrak JD, Hill NS, Federman EC, Kwa SL, O'Donnell C. Evaluation of intermittent long-term negative pressure ventilation in patients with severe obstructive pulmonary disease. *Am Rev Respir Dis* 1988;138:1515–8.
19 Kinnear WJM, Schneerson JM. Assisted ventilation in the home: is it worth considering? *Br J Dis Chest* 1985;79:313–51.
20 Shneerson JM. *Disorders of ventilation* Oxford: Blackwell, 1988.
21 Bach JR, Penek J. Obstructive sleep apnoea complicating negative-pressure ventilatory support in patients with chronic paralytic/restrictive ventilatory dysfunction. *Chest* 1991;99:1386–93.
22 Eve FG. Actuation of the inert diaphragm by a gravity method. *Lancet* 1932;ii:995–7.
23 Goldstein RS, Molotui N, Skrastins R, Long MS, Contreras M. Assisting ventilation in respiratory failure by negative pressure ventilation and by rocking bed. *Chest* 1987;92:470–4.
24 Judson JP, Glenn WWL. Radiofrequency electrophrenic respiration. Long-term application to a patient with primary hypoventilation. *JAMA* 1968;203:1033–7.
25 Liu HM, Loew JM, Hunt CE. Congenital hypoventilation syndrome: a pathologic study of the neuromuscular system. *Neurology* 1978;28:1013–9.
26 Moxham J, Schneerson JM. Diaphragmatic pacing. *Am Rev Respir Dis* 1993;148:533–6.

Index